16.95

AIDS: The HIV Myth

AIDS: The HIV Myth

Jad Adams

St. Martin's Press
New York

Library of Congress Cataloging-in-Publication Data

Adams, Jad.
          AIDS : the HIV myth.

              1. AIDS (Disease)—Etiology.   2. HIV (Viruses)
3. AIDS (Disease)—Research—Political aspects.
I. Title.
RC607.A26A3419   1989   616.97′92071   88-36238
ISBN 0-312-02859-8

First published in Great Britain by Macmillan London Limited.

First U.S. Edition

10 9 8 7 6 5 4 3 2 1

Contents

82792

Acknowledgments

Scientists too numerous to mention have assisted in aspects of work on this book. Most importantly Professor Gordon Stewart has examined drafts and given advice which has always been gratefully received.

Michael Verney-Elliott sowed the seed of my work on AIDS and without his persistence, his flying off at tangents and his relentless pursuit of exotic journal articles, the reasoning processes involved in this book would have been far less rewarding.

The support of David Lloyd and Karen Brown of *Dispatches* at Channel 4 television was essential to this work from the start, long may they continue to encourage journalism which considers there is more to a story than the repetition of government press releases.

Thanks to Joan Shenton at Meditel Productions, who made facilities available to me to work on this book.

Others who made contributions which did not result in their being quoted directly were: Felicity Milton at Meditel; Karen Hewitson and Paul Peakman for their help in Thailand; Amy Adams and Andrew Adams for their usual generous support.

Most of all, I must thank Julie Peakman, who helped throughout, including frequent late night discussions of Camus' *La Peste*, which the AIDS epidemic brings to mind for so many reasons.

Foreword

In 1960 a veteran retrovirologist urged his peers to 'raise questions whether the known facts about viruses suffice to account for it'. The subject was cancer, the veteran was Peyton Rous, and the quote is from a paper in *Cancer Research*. Mindful of that example, in 1987 I asked a similar question in a paper likewise published in *Cancer Research*: whether the known facts about two human retroviruses suffice to account for leukaemia and AIDS.

Clearly, following Rous's example did not make me very popular with the multinational club of retrovirologists. My article was officially ignored and not 'dignified' with a response because the AIDS virus establishment was 'too busy . . . saving lives' and testing for antibodies to HIV. I was often shunned like an AIDS patient by my former fellow retrovirologists. My views were unwelcome for several reasons: after a frustrating, twenty-year-long search for a human cancer virus, the retrovirologists were craving for clinical relevance and hence happily adopted HIV – 'the AIDS virus' – as the cause of AIDS. The discovery of HIV was announced in the US at a press conference and the virus-AIDS hypothesis became instant national dogma in the US. On this basis, the retrovirologists convinced their governments to spend billions of dollars to stop the predicted viral epidemic, already being labelled 'the epidemic of the 20th century'. The virus was also the immediate darling of the biotechnology companies. Due to its very low complexity, it can be readily cloned for diagnostic test kits and vaccines. In turn, the virus was a hit with the press because it mobilised in readers the instinctive fears of a contagious disease, and appealed to the public prejudice that all evil comes from without.

Even potential critics were infected by the AIDS viromania. Instead of criticising the virus, they were kept busy criticising virologists engaged in a three-year-long Franco-American legal battle over who first discovered the 'deadly virus'. Ironically, the fierce controversy generated further loyalties for the virus-AIDS hypothesis, since it would have been a farce if the battle had been fought over a virus that was not even the cause of AIDS.

Last summer, however, Jad Adams and his team from Meditel, Katie Leishman from the *Atlantic Monthly*, and John Lauritsen from the *New York Native* called for interviews – evidence for islands of common sense somewhere in the sea of AIDS viromania.

I am often asked why it is just myself, Harry Rubin, Joseph Sonnabend and a handful of others who question the virus-AIDS hypothesis. Why doesn't a young, ambitious scientist make a name for himself by questioning it? The answer lies in the strong conformist pressures on scientists, particularly young, untenured scientists, in the age of biotechnology. Their conceptual obedience to the establishment is maintained by controlled access to research grants, journals and positions, and rewarded by conference engagements, personal prizes, consultantships, stocks and co-ownership in companies. A dissenter would have to be truly independent and prepared for a variety of sanctions. I, for instance, was sarcastically called a 'brilliant chemist', but labelled a bigot for considering daily administration of psycho-active and immunosuppressive chemicals more likely to be the cause of AIDS than a chronically dormant and chemically almost undetectable retrovirus. Invitations were issued only on the condition that I did not debate the 'control' of AIDS with the AIDS test or the DNA-inhibitor AZT, both of which are based exclusively on the virus-AIDS hypothesis.

I hope that Jad Adams' book will not only entertain, but also open minds and free science to solve AIDS. Let me end with the words, again, of Peyton Rous: 'We are of many minds and opinions, yet we are one in the search for truth' (*Cancer Research*, 1960).

Peter Duesberg
Berkeley, California
20 July 1988

As opposed to its immediate predecessor, late twentieth-century science has given up all philosophical pretensions and has become a powerful business that shapes the mentality of its practitioners.

The most glorious achievements of the past are used not as instruments of enlightenment but as a means of intimidation . . . Let somebody make a great step forward – and the profession is bound to turn it into a club for beating people into submission.

Paul Feyerabend

One

Beginnings

THIS STORY STARTED, like all the best stories, with a routine procedure. Joan Shenton and I were television journalists working on medical and scientific programmes. As such we read the medical journals and kept a close watch on the curious events of the 1980s.

We had no call to do any work on AIDS but we knew the big events: a new disease discovered infecting homosexuals in 1981; proposals that it was caused by a virus, perhaps even a new kind called a retrovirus, in 1982; a retrovirus discovered by the French in 1983; and by the Americans in 1984; three years spent arguing over who got there first; increasingly febrile threats of a heterosexual epidemic; persecution of homosexuals.

There is enough in that to make any half-way cynical hack raise an eyebrow but my suspicious nature was mollified by the knowledge that there was a story of scientific fraud which was already receiving sufficient coverage. I didn't think there was anything for us in it.

That was when the routine procedure came in. Joan, who runs Meditel Productions, and I felt it almost a public duty to see people who said they had a story. We were supposed to be investigative journalists but we were making programmes out of a genuine public-spiritedness, as well as the joy of the chase. We saw all comers: the Czech émigré who found the secret of the universe in carefully drawn geometrical formulae; the doleful warehouseman who wanted to do a documentary on hands; the actress who wanted to describe the social isolation of albinos; the archaeologist who wanted to make his subject accessible to a popular audience; the Australian girl who favoured a documentary on farting. Somewhere I have a file.

Michael Verney-Elliott was one of these who had a story. I was immediately suspicious when I knew it was about AIDS: ever since the first homosexuals had gone down with the disease speculation on it had been the preserve of loonies and conspiracy theorists.

Michael's charm and humour dispelled most fears that this was a crazy hoping to air paranoid delusions in public. He sat before us – quick, dark-haired, looking much younger than forty-nine, witty, bitchy, camp and overwhelmingly informative.

Too informative. Like most people with an enthusiasm, he wanted to get it all out at once. Michael presented us with the difficult task of collecting tiny nuggets of usable fact from the torrent of information. Most importantly, he asked questions which begged to be answered: If AIDS began in Africa, why did it spread first to America rather than Europe where we have far closer links with Africa?

Why are AIDS victims dying of sheep diseases and bird diseases which we'd never heard of before, rather than more common human diseases? Why die of Pneumocystis carinii pneumonia when you can die from ordinary pulmonary pneumonia?

If women can get AIDS as easily as men, where are all the dead women? Have they given up semen?

Why has some of the most promising work, like that connecting AIDS with African swine fever virus, just been discarded?

If AIDS is caused by a virus called HIV, why has HIV never been found in Factor VIII which is what is supposed to have infected the haemophiliacs?

What was the role of the plasma dealers in spreading infected blood products around the world?

At least some of these questions could form the basis of an exciting investigative programme. It was time to open another bottle of wine and write out an application for some research funding.

This book is not about how to make a television programme, and the complex details of research and filming in different countries would be a fruitless distraction. There were the usual problems with a large project: nail-biting impatience for funding, work late into the night, jet lag, short-tempered arguments with other staff, being let down by erstwhile supporters and finding encouragement in unexpected places.

Michael established himself in a corner of the office surrounded by scientific journals and with a constant infusion of black coffee. His chain smoking and his explosions of enthusiasm made daily life with Michael rather like keeping a small volcano as a house guest.

Michael was a tonic against idleness – he would not allow propositions to go unchallenged. When we started out I did not even accept, until I had seen the proof of it, that AIDS is a condition which can be transmitted from one person to another. If there were prizes for honest doubt, we deserved them.

After months of research and hundreds of hours of reasoning we came to the conclusion that the theory that HIV causes AIDS was either wrong or severely deficient. Let me repeat that: the theory that a retrovirus called human immunodeficiency virus causes AIDS after a long latency period in up to one hundred per cent of infected people just does not fit the facts of the AIDS epidemic.

We had come to this conclusion before March 1987 when a devastating critique of the theory that HIV causes AIDS was published in the journal *Cancer Research*. Its author, Professor Peter Duesberg from Berkeley, was one of the world's leading retrovirologists. His deductive method of reasoning was refreshing after dealing for so long with scientists who expected their view to be taken as an article of faith. When science cannot be questioned it is not science any more, it is religion. Duesberg was a scientist after our own hearts, he made deductions based on known facts and when he did not know something he said so. There are limitations to the deductive method, however. It is better at criticising existing theories than founding new ones. It is possible to say HIV does not cause AIDS, based on the evidence designed to prove it does. It is not possible, from that evidence, to prove what does cause AIDS.

We looked at the four groups who formed the so-called 4H club of infected people at the start of the epidemic: homosexuals, heroin users, haemophiliacs and Haitians. What predisposed them to develop AIDS so quickly when the 'heterosexual epidemic' which has been threatened for so long has been taking its time in coming?

Once one brick had been removed from the edifice of a theory about the cause and spread of AIDS, it was remarkably easy to dislodge the rest. Notions about the extent of AIDS – the view that there are ten million carriers in the world, for example – are largely based on evidence from Africa which would be unacceptable in an undergraduate essay if it referred to Western disease patterns.

Ideas about the origin of AIDS have been dismissed as crazy only in order for supporters of the equally crazy theory of a monkey origin of the disease to enjoy precedence.

The image of zealous researchers confronting AIDS as a new problem and by superhuman effort finding the cause in a matter of months verges on the comic. The story of AIDS is deeply connected with the vicissitudes of the theory that viruses cause cancer and the failure of the cancer research programme. Michael put it most acidly when he said: 'From the people who didn't bring you the virus which causes cancer, it's the virus that doesn't cause AIDS.'

Theories rise and fall in scientific research much as they do in any other arena. Debates are won by the most eloquent, by those with the most financial clout, by those with friends in the appropriate places. Nothing demonstrates this so well as the AIDS story.

The pace at which the politics and financing of the AIDS industry proceeded in the early nineteen-eighties meant that caution was thrown to the winds. Theory was piled on supposition about AIDS, hyperbole was piled on hyperbole. Dissenting voices were unheard: drowned out or deliberately silenced.

It is perfectly clear, as the heterosexual epidemic fails to occur to any great degree, that serious mistakes were made in AIDS research. Action was taken on those mistaken beliefs and it has benefited some interest groups at the expense of others.

The cause of AIDS is still not understood but some of the theories of its cause – in particular of the part syphilis is said to play in its development – shed light on the disease and provide information about treatment which is not forthcoming from the theory that HIV causes AIDS.

Part of the reason why a newly discovered virus like HIV could be misidentified as the cause of a complex syndrome like AIDS is that all the fields of research involved in the AIDS story are themselves complex and no individual scientist has an adequate command of all of them, each having to rely on the insights and choices made by specialists in other fields in order to corroborate from other disciplines the insights of one particular speciality. Thus the epidemiologist, who studies epidemics, is obliged to believe in the choices made by the virologist, who studies viruses, and vice versa; neither will have sufficient command of the other's discipline to be capable of judgement, particularly when the other discipline is straining past the point of knowledge and into speculation as has so often been the case in the AIDS story.

The major disciplines making up the AIDS story are virology and molecular biology; immunology (the study of the immune system); pathology (the study of disease states); the social sciences and epidemiology. This book attempts to give adequate information in these disciplines to render the AIDS story accessible to a general reader. It is hoped that no disservice is done to the truth in the process of simplification.

One problem with the judgement of science is that its jargon tends to separate it from public scrutiny. Lay people do not feel confident about making even the most commonsense observations on scientific subjects if they do not know the correct jargon. The jargon indeed confuses but the concepts involved in scientific papers – particularly in the biological sciences – are not difficult to grasp. I am attempting here to approach the subject-matter with as little jargon as possible.

I see no need to apologise for the subjective style in which this book is written. As part of its intention is to demonstrate how the scientific observer selects and alters that which is observed, it would be churlish of this literary observer to pretend to objectivity.

Two

Patients

New York

JOE SONNABEND STRETCHED in his battered leather chair and rubbed his eyes. It was the end of another day running a surgery in Greenwich Village. Most of his patients were gays and most of their problems were related to lifestyle: venereal diseases, bowel parasites, sports injuries. They were mainly healthy young men with sporadic problems which could be treated successfully.

That last patient had been odd, though. Raised purplish blotches over the skin of his legs and trunk. Had had them for some months and expected them to go away on their own. Very strange.

Joe suddenly got up and went to the brown patient files. Hadn't he seen that before? Yes, three months before, that slight blond man from Charles Street. It had just affected his feet, and it was more embarrassing to him than anything else.

The curious doctor had reached for a medical textbook. He had made a tentative diagnosis of Kaposi's sarcoma. The book read: 'A malignant, multifocal neoplasm of reticuloendothelial cells that begins as soft, brownish or purple papules on the feet and slowly spreads in the skin, metastasising to the lymph nodes and viscera.'

But it was a disease of the elderly – old Jewish and Italian men got it and died of cancer or heart disease or some other condition long before the slowly developing skin lesions could cause a problem.

Joe wasn't a native New Yorker, he came from Africa where they had a similar disease. Kaposi's sarcoma in young people. Two cases in New York in a few months. Wonder if there were any more, perhaps he would call some colleagues who were also in general practice to see if they could shed any light on it. As Joe left his surgery that night, he had a bad feeling in the pit of his stomach.

Los Angeles

Christmas 1980 is when the AIDS story is normally said to begin, at the University of California at Los Angeles where work at the School of Medicine was winding down for the festive season.

Immunologist Michael Gottlieb was called by a colleague to see a thirty-one-year-old white man with a leukaemia diagnosis. The most obvious sign of illness, however, was Candida albicans, a yeast infection commonly known as thrush which is often found in the mouths and vaginas of the sexually active but which is never found in young people in so great a quantity as in this patient.

Arnold, a Los Angeles artist and a homosexual who had never been sick before, was choking with it. His throat was blocked by the fluffy white growth. Gottlieb had access to the latest technology because a colleague was doing research work with it. The new equipment was used to count Arnold's T cells.

The reason for this is that the T cells are supposed to hold back minor infections. Gottlieb judged that if there was a problem of otherwise petty infections becoming serious, it must have its root in the T cells.

The cell counter found a major depletion of T helper cells, an integral part of the immune system. Arnold soon developed a severe pneumonia. An open lung biopsy, a technique not usually performed on seriously ill patients, disclosed Pneumocystis carinii pneumonia, a rare disease caused by a protozoan parasite. He did not live long. Christmas 1980 was the last Merry Christmas for the homosexual community in American cities.

By May 1981 Michael Gottlieb and colleagues he had contacted to discuss the phenomenon treated five young homosexuals with Pneumocystis carinii pneumonia and other opportunistic infections. They reported the cases in the 5 June 1981 issue of the *Morbidity and Mortality Weekly Report* published by the Centers for Disease Control in Atlanta, Georgia, in order to keep doctors up to date with current health problems and statistics.

Opportunistic infections in people with immune dysfunction are not remarkable, of course. If they were, then physicians would never have been able to identify them in these new patients. In fact no single infection apparent in AIDS at this time was new. What was new in the early nineteen-eighties was their appearance in individuals who were otherwise healthy.

The infections

Life-threatening opportunistic infections would normally be seen in those suffering from malnutrition in the Third World or, in technologically advanced countries, in organ transplant patients whose immune system would have been broken down with drugs to assist in acceptance of the new organ. It would otherwise have been rejected by the immune system as a foreign invader.

Though generally healthy, Joe Sonnabend's patients had always presented with illnesses which were rather different from those a general practitioner would normally expect to see.

'I was seeing patients with a whole range of problems for years before AIDS came along,' he said.

Swollen lymph glands, bladder problems, bowel problems of course. I was telling them this was going to lead to some major problem though I didn't know what. People would come in for treatment for gonorrhoea, get their shot of penicillin and go straight back to the bath houses to have sex again. They'd do that ten times a year. Of course there were going to be problems. One of my promiscuous patients would already have hepatitis B, hepatitis A, syphilis, gonorrhoea, cytomegalovirus, herpes simplex, Epstein-Barr virus. It is not a moralistic point to tell people they are running into trouble if they are doing things which will leave them harbouring all these infections, it is a medical point.

Most of the infections which rack the bodies of AIDS patients were already present in those bodies when the men were healthy. The immune system was keeping them at bay. It was possible to tell that the AIDS patients had some serious, unusual problem because they were suffering from the unusual conditions Kaposi's sarcoma and Pneumocystis carinii pneumonia. People without AIDS or immune deficiency may suffer seriously from herpes or hepatitis B, but an otherwise apparently healthy young man is extremely unlikely to suffer from Pneumocystis or Kaposi's unless he has AIDS.

This issue is central to the question of whether HIV is the cause of the disease. HIV could be just another one of the many infections being passed around by those at 'high risk' of developing AIDS. In the absence of a functioning immune system, otherwise harmless or controllable infections run riot.

The following does not claim to be anything like a complete description of the conditions of AIDS patients. Probably some of the infections which AIDS patients have are caused by micro-organisms which have not been described; they do not even figure in the textbooks.

It is important to remember, in the light of the question of whether HIV causes AIDS, that HIV is one micro-organism in a thronging menagerie.

Some of the conditions of AIDS patients, notably Kaposi's sarcoma, are not believed even to be infectious.

Kaposi's sarcoma

Several of the early reports of Kaposi's sarcoma in young men in New York were referred to Alvin Friedman-Kien, Professor of Dermatology at New York University. He had, he estimated, seen thirty cases of Kaposi's sarcoma in his life, all in elderly men. Now he had heard of almost that number in a year and all in young homosexuals. He reported the cases in the CDC's *Morbidity and Mortality Weekly Report* for 3 July 1981. It was about this point that cases stopped being counted in ones and twos and started being numbered in scores. In a year it was to be hundreds, then thousands. Hungarian dermatologist Moriz Kaposi could never have guessed how famous he was to become more than a century after he first described Kaposi's sarcoma when looking for external signs of syphilis in 1872. Classical Kaposi's sarcoma is a skin cancer affecting elderly men of Ashkenazi Jewish or Mediterranean Italian background. It starts as one or two small, raised red or purple patches. These grow, over a period of ten to fifteen years, until they cover the surface of the lower legs. There is also an aggressive variety of KS seen in Africa, particularly sub-Saharan Africa, which affects young adults.

AIDS Kaposi's sarcoma may affect any area of skin as well as internal organs. New lesions develop quickly over a period of weeks or months. Normally KS itself does not threaten life though occasionally concomitant diseases of the abdomen and lungs produce heavy bleeding from the KS lesions which may prove lethal. Localised sarcoma can affect the head and become cosmetically distressing. These can be treated with radiation like other tumours. Bleeding lesions on the feet, penis and mouth can also be treated with radiation.

Unusually aggressive KS is also found in kidney transplant patients whose immune system has been suppressed by drugs. If immuno-suppression stops, the disease diminishes. About one-third of these patients die of KS rather than kidney failure or infection.

For a reason not fully understood, while half of all homosexual AIDS cases get KS, only ten per cent of IV drug users or Haitian AIDS patients do. Very few cases have been reported in haemophiliacs.

Heredity has been suggested as one reason for this: as KS is classically found in Italian and Jewish men, this must mean there is a genetic predisposition to develop this tumour throughout the whole of these men's lives. Perhaps the homosexual patients with KS were Jewish or Italian – perhaps some environmental factor in Jewish or Italian families predisposed boys to become homosexuals. Unfortunately for researchers working on this theory, while once there were high figures recorded for KS AIDS patients also having particular Jewish or Italian genetic markers, as time has gone on and more studies have been performed, these figures have dropped. In some studies the level of Jewish or Italian genetic markers has been no higher than in the general population.

It is interesting that KS is endemic in Equatorial Africa where Epstein-Barr virus, found in nearly all homosexual AIDS patients if not all of them, is also endemic. Epstein-Barr virus is probably responsible for Burkitt's lymphoma, almost the only human cancer to have been found with a likely viral origin.

Some explanation is required for the use of so many conditional terms – 'almost', 'probable', 'likely'. Surely it is or it isn't? Alas, no. These are the facts as related by Alan Cantwell:

> Most scientists now believe Epstein-Barr virus causes Burkitt's lymphoma. However, this has not been proven. Over eighty per cent of healthy, normal, black African children under the age of five years carry the virus. As many as twenty per cent of the tumours occurring in Africa do not show evidence of the virus. It is possible the virus may only reside as a 'passenger' in the tumour tissue. Only fifteen to twenty per cent of Burkitt's lymphoma tumours found elsewhere in the world contain Epstein-Barr virus. Two of three tumours tested in San Francisco patients contained Epstein-Barr virus antigens. One tumour also contained cytomegalovirus antigens.

It is possible for honourable and respected medical scientists to hold exactly contrary views based on different interpretations of the same facts. The facts quoted above 'prove' that Burkitt's lymphoma is caused by Epstein-Barr virus. They also 'prove' the opposite. In all the really important debates, medical science is as exact as literature.

Researchers have found cytomegalovirus in the lesions of Kaposi's sarcoma. Cytomegalo is another of the viruses found in almost one hundred per cent of homosexual men with AIDS. Unfortunately this track, like the Epstein-Barr virus connection, has led nowhere.

It has been suggested that repeated infections with cytomegalovirus in genetically predisposed persons who have an immune disbalance will cause Kaposi's sarcoma. This is, of course, only a suggestion as to what ingredients in which order might produce this one manifestation of AIDS. The biological pathways by which this could occur are not understood.

It has been suggested that Kaposi's sarcoma is AIDS. This view takes the standpoint that KS is apparent in all AIDS cases, though in an underlying inflammatory form in patients who do not have the characteristic lesions. Like many other promising ideas, this one failed to attract research effort after HIV was declared the cause.

Alan Cantwell, a Los Angeles dermatologist, believes in the theory that a so-called 'pleomorphic' bacteria – one which passes through several stages in which it changes its shape – is responsible for causing cancer, including Kaposi's sarcoma. He says he has identified such a microbe in lesions of Kaposi's sarcoma. 'Could it be possible,' he writes, 'that scientists have been overlooking important bacteriologic findings in AIDS, by concentrating heavily on the virus theory of AIDS?'

To restate this: AIDS was very quickly reckoned to be caused by a virus. Viruses are not complete organisms which can live independently of their host. They need to live in the body cells of living things. Viruses are small, even in terms of microbiology. Antibiotics, like penicillin, do not work against viruses.

Bacteria are much larger and they are whole organisms which may live some or all of their time outside an animal. They are killed by antibiotics.

Alan Cantwell's case is that AIDS may be caused by a bacteria and that the pursuit of the virus before other possible causes of AIDS were fully examined meant that evidence pointing to a bacterial origin of AIDS was overlooked.

To say Cantwell's view is a minority one is to overstate it. He may be in a minority of one. He is interesting, however, because he is a scientist with adequate access to all the information who derives from that information quite different conclusions from those favoured by the 'AIDS establishment', who promote the hypothesis that HIV causes AIDS. This is a situation we encounter repeatedly in the AIDS story.

In order to understand some part of the complexity of what is happening in an AIDS patient's body it is helpful for the reader to have some acquaintance with the micro-organisms which are most frequently found there. This list is far from exhaustive.

Pneumocystis carinii and other protozoa

The patient who presented to his doctor in Greenwich Village with Kaposi's sarcoma will have found this only the most obvious manifestation of his illness, the one most certainly requiring medical attention.

The first indication that something was wrong would have been fever, chills and drenching night sweats. He would have suffered unexplained fatigue lasting weeks, a weight loss of ten or more pounds in less than two months, persistent diarrhoea.

Lymph node enlargement – lymphadenopathy – may indicate AIDS or it may mean the body is defending itself against some other problem. The lymph nodes in the neck and groin often become swollen as a reaction to a variety of infections.

Many early symptoms of AIDS patients could be caused by a wide variety of factors: bruising, excessive bleeding, headaches and depression. The symptom most likely to cause a patient to go to a doctor in the absence of Kaposi's sarcoma is shortness of breath. This is caused by infection by Pneumocystis carinii. This is a single-celled organism – its body comprises of one cell, unlike more complex animals like ourselves which are made up of many millions of cells. These simplest creatures of the animal kingdom are called protozoa. Because they are animals they are considered to be parasites, just as lice are. It would not be an abuse of language to refer to all micro-organisms infesting a body as parasites but generally the term is used only of other animals.

For most of this century parasitic diseases had been dismissed as curiosities of 'tropical medicine'; people in rich countries did not die of such things.

Now this normally harmless parasite, which many if not all healthy people carry about with them, has become the major immediate cause of death in AIDS patients.

The organism was first described in 1909 but not identified as a cause of human illness until 1951. In the US the first adult case was observed in 1954. Until AIDS almost all cases in America were severely ill patients undergoing cancer chemotherapy or organ transplants – both causes of immune depression. Around the world, the majority of pneumocystis deaths are in children in the Third World who are immune deficient because of malnutrition. Cases among German infants in the late nineteen-thirties were retrospectively diagnosed as Pneumocystis carinii.

The organism replicates in the lung until by sheer bulk it irritates the lining of the lung and provokes inflammation. In the patient the evidence for this is in breathing difficulties – he cannot get sufficient oxygen into his blood because of the inflammation of his lungs. For a reason not understood, there is a correlation between the incidence of pneumocystis and of eye defects in AIDS patients. It is possible that the parasite is invading other organs, including the eye.

A patient who first presents with KS can expect to live around two years. A patient whose first medically treated symptom of AIDS is pneumocystis will have around one year to live.

In terms of size, the protozoa are the largest micro-organisms to infect AIDS victims. Next come fungi, bacteria and then viruses. This is a general rule and many organisms stubbornly refuse to obey it. There is variation over the size categories and behaviour patterns.

Toxoplasma gondii: another usually harmless protozoan, which is devastating in patients with damaged immune systems. It too can cause pneumonia. It can also be responsible for damage to the heart muscle but its most devastating effect is on the brain, where it causes inflammation leading to confusion, dizziness, seizures and death.

Cryptosporidium: this has only recently been known to infect humans. Dr Kevin Cahill from the Tropical Disease Center, New York, notes that 'Less than a decade ago it was recognised solely in turkeys, snakes, calves, lambs and various rodents.' It had been found to infect vets who came into contact with infected animals with a mild, self-limiting diarrhoea. In AIDS patients, however, the diarrhoea is torrential. Dr Cahill writes: 'A daily loss of almost twenty litres of diarrhoeal fluid was seen in one AIDS victim for whom I consulted.'

Dr Cahill also notes that the island of Manhattan has become well-known as a focus for tropical infections. He is referring to the 'gay bowel syndrome' or 'bath house syndrome'. This was a feature of medical practice in homosexual areas for a decade before the outbreak of AIDS and consists of the intestinal parasites which are common in parts of the world where hygiene and standards of food preparation are poor – Entameba histolytica causing amoebiasis and Giardia lamblia causing giardiasis. These are among the deadliest diseases in the world, in that diarrhoea is the major cause of childhood death and these are diarrhoeal diseases, though they are far from being the only ones or the most virulent.

Fungi

The diseases caused by fungi are minor irritations in immunocompetent humans – those with an intact and functioning immune system.

The most common fungal infection seen in AIDS patients is caused by a yeast, a single-cell fungus. Candida albicans coats the mouth and throat with thick, white plaques.

Cryptococcus enters via the lungs and spreads to other organs, causing severe meningitis in the brain. Histoplasma, Coccidiodes and Blastomyces are other fungi which can be recovered from AIDS patients.

Bacteria

Tuberculosis is another disease of poverty which has been brought to the fore by AIDS. Mycobacterium tuberculosis produces small lumps in any part of the body but normally in the lung. The disease causes coughing, emaciation and eventually death.

Classical tuberculosis is, of course, a common disease among people who are not AIDS patients or immune-suppressed so it is not one of the 'opportunistic infections' characteristic of AIDS.

Mycobacterium avium-intercellulare causes other forms of tuberculosis and it is decidedly opportunistic, seen previously only in elderly men with diseases which suppressed their immune systems. The bacteria is found in soil, water and house dust. The infections spread beyond the lung to the major organs including the brain.

Other bacteria found in AIDS patients are Salmonella causing intestinal inflammation; Salmonella typhii causing typhoid fever; the Nocardia soil bacteria causing lung disease; Listeria monocytogenes causing a severe brain infection.

AIDS patients are also more prone than the general population to pneumonias caused by bacteria and to common hospital-acquired infections.

Chlamydia trachomatis is one of those micro-organisms which is difficult to classify. It has its own cell wall, like the bacteria, but is dependent on its host cell, like the viruses. Its dependence is that it cannot itself synthesise adenosine triphosphate (ATP) which is essential for movement, so it must take this from the cell it inhabits. It is sexually transmitted and infects both men and women, causing 'slow burn' inflammatory diseases of the urethra (the urinary tube) in men. In women it causes inflammation of the cervix and pelvic inflammatory disease. It is the commonest sexually transmitted disease in urban populations of developing and developed countries.

Perhaps the most important bacterium to infect AIDS patients is Treponema pallidum, the spiral-shaped organism which causes syphilis. Antibodies against syphilis are found in up to seventy per cent of AIDS patients but the literature on syphilis always warns that 'false negative' results – those indicating a patient is not infected when in fact he is – can occur if the disease is in a latent phase or if the patient's immune system is not functioning normally. Syphilis in its late form (tertiary syphilis) sees the bacteria invading any cell of the body and damaging any organ of the body. Syphilis will be dealt with in detail later as it is probable that it plays a far greater part in AIDS than has generally been recognised.

Viral infections

AIDS had almost from the start been felt to be an infectious disease because of its spread – from homosexual to homosexual, from drug addict to drug addict, from blood supply to haemophiliac, from Haitian to Haitian. Of course, there are reasons why these groups are immune-suppressed and it is possible that the opportunistic infections of AIDS were simply occurring in immune-suppressed people as they had in, for example, kidney transplant patients, long before the AIDS epidemic.

The four risk groups will be examined in detail later. The point in this context is that an infectious agent was sought. What kind of an agent? A virus was suspected largely for reasons rooted in recent history. For twenty years cancer researchers had tried to identify viruses which caused cancer. Their success had been limited, to put it mildly, but by 1980 it seemed likely that Epstein-Barr virus was responsible for two minor cancers (minor in terms of the number of people they affected) and cytomegalovirus had been found to cause T-cell deficiencies in man and animals. Both were found in AIDS patients.

Viruses are small, even compared to bacteria. Where bacteria are complete organisms, living in an almost parasitic relationship with man and other animals, viruses cannot be considered to have an existence separate from their host. Viruses are genetic programmes which connect to cells in a living organism and use that cell's own structure to replicate.

The viruses most characteristic of AIDS are herpes viruses, specifically cytomegalo, Epstein-Barr, herpes simplex types I and II and varicella zoster. Herpes viruses remain latent for long periods until triggered off by some event in the body including immunosuppression.

Cytomegalovirus is excreted in the saliva and semen of many homosexuals with AIDS. Antibodies to it are widespread and are found in all or almost all AIDS patients. Cytomegalo on first infection causes a suppression of the immune system which may last for weeks or months. This is accompanied by fever, lymph node enlargement and fatigue. Several viruses, it will be seen, can cause these conditions which are characteristic of the very first stages of AIDS.

People in high-risk categories, and particularly promiscuous homosexuals, will have been re-infected with cytomegalo several times. After the initial illness, there will be no symptoms. The virus resides in the kidneys and uro-genital tract and infects the endothelial cells which line blood vessels. This has been noted as possibly having a special significance in AIDS because Kaposi's sarcoma involves endothelial cells and parts of cytomegalo have been found in KS lesions.

Cytomegalo infection has been a major problem in transplant recipients, immune suppressed because of the drugs they are taking to prevent rejection of the new organ, and in babies congenitally infected with it. These babies, whose immune systems will be undeveloped, are said to resemble babies with AIDS.

In AIDS patients the cytomegalo can cause pneumonia, where it can co-exist in the lung with Pneumocystis carinii. It can also cause colitis (inflammation of the bowel); retinitis (inflammation of the retina) leading to blindness; encephalitis (inflammation of the brain) and abnormalities in the functioning of the liver.

Cytomegalo has long been thought to play a primary role in AIDS and has been seriously considered as a candidate for the cause. Cytomegalo was obviously there in the disease. The question asked in the early days was: Is it in the driving seat or the passenger seat? It is spread in semen and blood, it can cause immune suppression, albeit transiently, and antibodies to it are found in most AIDS patients. The reason why most researchers rejected it as a cause is because it has been present in humans for a long time without causing epidemic illness; it is found in people without AIDS as well as people with AIDS, and because there was no peculiar genetic structure to strains of cytomegalo which did not occur in AIDS patients as compared to those which did.

All these criticisms could, of course, be levelled against HIV which is generally believed to be the cause of AIDS. As will be examined, the reason why these perfectly common-sense arguments prevailed against cytomegalo as the cause but not against HIV is more rooted in the politics of science than in the logic of it.

Genital herpes was the sexually transmitted plague which preceded AIDS. Herpes simplex II is the second most common viral infection in patients with AIDS. This is hardly surprising considering the sexual lifestyle of most people at risk for AIDS and the fact that, in the US for example, an estimated twenty million people have it. Herpes appears as painful, raised pustules on the genitals. The virus resides in the nerve cells of the host until it is activated by changes in the body – including lowered immunity.

For this reason AIDS patients suffer frequent episodes of viral reactivation and the spread of the herpes lesions, uncontrolled by the immune system as they are in healthy people, is extensive. Patients may develop perianal ulcers which expand to several inches in diameter and will not regress.

Herpes simplex I is commonly known as the virus which causes cold sores. These affect twenty per cent of the population of the UK and twenty to forty per cent in the US.

The pustules are similar in appearance to those which infect the genitals and it has been suggested that it is the same virus, mutated into a slightly different strain, which was spread from mouth to genitals by oro-genital contact.

'Cold sores' appear on the lips and face and are contained by the immune system after they have erupted. AIDS patients therefore suffer uncontrolled outbreaks on the face which result in gaping ulcers.

The herpesviruses are not destroyed by the immune system – though almost one hundred per cent of homosexuals have antibodies to them whether or not they have AIDS – because their long periods of latency are spent in the nerve cells which are beyond the influence of the immune system. They spark an antibody response when they travel down the nerve cells to the skin and the infected skin cells summon the immune system.

Reinfection with mutating herpes may produce more serious illness than the initial infection, if the animal studies are to be believed. In a laboratory study mice were infected with two different strains of herpesvirus, neither of which was lethal to mice. Two-thirds of the mice died and eleven variant strains of the two original strains were isolated. Three of these were invariably lethal to mice. A new lethal strain had been developed by the interaction of different non-lethal strains of the virus. Is it possible that this happened in the bodies of AIDS victims who were constantly exposed to new strains of viruses including herpesviruses?

Another virus common to almost all AIDS patients is Epstein-Barr. It is the most common cause of infectious mononucleosis, also called 'kissing disease' and 'glandular fever'. This is characterised by transient depression of the immune system, headache, sore throat, mental and physical fatigue, weakness and enlarged lymph nodes. These symptoms are, of course, characteristic of the first stages of AIDS. They are also the sign of infection with cytomegalovirus which is often associated with infectious mononucleosis.

Another common name for infectious mononucleosis is 'student's disease' because of the lifestyle of students which predisposes them to develop it. The typical patient in this case is a student who is working hard, late into the night and so suffering fatigue without enjoying the compensation of sleep. The student will be eating poorly both through poverty and, more likely, an inability to appreciate nutritional needs. The patient is also likely to be sexually active, perhaps promiscuously so, and is likely to contract the infection from a partner's saliva.

Epstein-Barr virus enjoys a remarkable position in that it is one of only a small number of viruses which have been closely implicated as probable causes of human cancers. In the case of Epstein-Barr, two cancers are said to be caused in some cases of infection: nasopharyngeal cancer and Burkitt's lymphoma. In the case of Burkitt's lymphoma there is a connection with AIDS in that malignant lymphoma, very similar to Burkitt's, is the most common tumour in AIDS patients after Kaposi's sarcoma. It affects the lymph nodes, resulting most obviously in an egg-like swelling on the neck. It is aggressive in AIDS patients and unresponsive to treatment, usually attacking lymph nodes, bone marrow and brain membranes. The average survival rate for AIDS patients after developing malignant lymphoma is one year.

Its relationship with the immune system and its frequency in AIDS patients has led some people to believe Epstein-Barr virus has a strongly contributive, if not causative, role in AIDS.

Varicella zoster virus is the last of the herpesviruses to be considered here. In children it is known as chicken pox where it is a mild illness involving fever and a rash. The virus will have been inhaled, spread from the throat to the lymphatic system then carried to the skin where blisters appear.

In adults a first infection of chicken pox is much more severe than in children and shingles, a reactivation of Varicella zoster virus, appears frequently in the elderly and the immunocompromised. Shingles, known as herpes zoster, is an agonisingly painful condition characterised by a series of blisters around the trunk, the 'belt of fire'. It is common in AIDS patients.

Antibodies to hepatitis A virus have been found in eighty-six per cent of homosexual AIDS patients. It is a common disease causing inflammation of the liver, as its name suggests. It is transmitted through contaminated food or water and is most common in children.

Hepatitis B is entirely different except in that it also infects the liver, though in the case of this virus the disease is far more severe. Hepatitis B is transmitted by infected blood and blood products, the sharing of contaminated syringes by drug addicts, infected semen and saliva. When the virus reaches the liver it causes functional damage which may be irreversible. Up to ninety-four per cent of homosexual AIDS patients have been found to have antibodies to hepatitis B virus.

Concentrations of antibodies against hepatitis B virus are so high in some homosexuals that homosexuals contributed towards a plasma collection scheme aimed at fighting the virus in those newly infected with it. In a display of public-spiritedness which said much for the morale among the homosexual community in the immediately pre-AIDS period, men queued up to donate plasma from which was made hepatitis B-immune globulin which was available to treat health workers who had become accidentally exposed to hepatitis B while handling infected blood.

Another product of this campaign using the high levels of hepatitis B in some homosexuals for the benefit of all at-risk people was the production of hepatitis B vaccine obtained by taking the virus from hepatitis B carriers, killing it and injecting it into the uninfected to induce them to produce their own antibody protection.

Ironically, after the beginning of the AIDS epidemic, suspicion surrounded these protections against hepatitis B because of the role of homosexuals in their production. In fact no gamma globulin, including hepatitis B-immune globulin, has been associated with AIDS.

Papovaviruses cause warts in the general population. They belong to a varied group which includes human papilloma virus 16, another one of the few viruses which have been implicated in human cancer – in this case cervical cancer, which is probably not involved in AIDS.

The majority of people, both healthy and with AIDS, who are tested for antibody towards papovaviruses show up positive. One of these viruses is claimed to be responsible for progressive multifocal leukoencephalopathy which causes loss of memory, inability to concentrate, motor function failure and depression. Some autopsies have failed to find viral particles in the brain of patients who have died with this condition which leaves a question mark over whether or not it is a viral disease at all. Papovaviruses may all be harmless passengers.

Around thirty-five different types of human *adenoviruses* are known to exist, usually passengers causing no problems. They do cause respiratory infections and lymphadenopathy but rarely lead to serious illness in otherwise healthy adults. Even in AIDS patients these infections are rarely lethal, though immunosuppressed bone marrow transplant patients have suffered from disease due to disseminated adenovirus infection.

The virus which after many arguments over terminology came to be termed Human Immunodeficiency Virus (HIV) is sometimes referred to as 'the AIDS virus' because it is believed to be the cause of AIDS. This claim, and the way in which it came to be made, is the subject of this book, so only the main facts about this virus need to be mentioned here. It was discovered in 1983 in tissue taken from a patient suffering from swollen lymph glands. It is known to infect T4 cells but, in common with other viruses mentioned here, both pathogenic and non-pathogenic, it is also disseminated throughout many other parts of the body – it has been found in macrophages, Langerhans' cells and brain cells. On initial infection it is known to cause a mononucleosis-like temporary condition in common with cytomegalo and Epstein-Barr viruses. It is spread through contact with infected blood, blood products and semen. In this it resembles hepatitis B virus but it is still a matter for discussion whether it is possible to contract HIV from contaminated saliva. Up to ninety per cent of AIDS patients have antibodies to HIV.

Human B Cell Lymphotropic virus was isolated from AIDS patients in 1986. It is present in at least fifty per cent of AIDS patients but also thirty per cent of healthy individuals. It is not known if it is pathogenic. It is now known as Human herpes virus six, HHV6.

Two other viruses may be mentioned here, African Swine Fever virus which was reported to be found in the blood of a high proportion of AIDS patients and a 'novel virus' which was reported by Shyh-Ching Lo to have been identified from an AIDS patient in 1986.

The Fourth International Conference on AIDS in Stockholm in June 1988 found Dr Lo, of the Armed Forces Institute of Pathology, Washington, giving two abstracts about his discovery which he had now designated a 'virus-like infectious agent' rather than a true virus. This agent, VLIA-sb51, was isolated from an AIDS patient, grown in a cell line and used to infect four monkeys. 'All four infected monkeys showed wasting syndromes, transient lymphadenopathy, and died in 7–9 months.'

This information caused great excitement among the community which questions whether HIV is the cause of AIDS. Here Lo had fulfilled two of the criteria for demonstrating that an infectious agent causes a disease – he had recovered the agent from an AIDS patient and had infected susceptible laboratory animals with it which then suffered something close to the original disease. This is a good deal more than has been achieved with HIV.

Caution is the best policy, however. The experimental monkeys used did show a weakened antibody response, which implies the immune system was disrupted by the agent, but they did not show the opportunistic infections characteristic of AIDS. It could be that VLIA-sb51 is just another of the opportunistic infections colonising immune-suppressed AIDS patients.

To be considered as a candidate for the cause of AIDS this agent would first have to be found in many AIDS patients. It would, of course, have to be sought before it was found and this is the difficulty the preoccupation with HIV has caused for those who feel it most appropriate to retain an open mind on the subject of the cause of AIDS – little work is being done on other candidates.

Shyh-Ching Lo enjoys some protection from the US 'AIDS establishment' which promotes HIV as the sole cause of AIDS because he works for the military rather than the government-funded health institutions.

The above should give some indication of the range of the microbiological zoo infesting AIDS patients. The cause may be one of them, or it may be none of them, or it could be a combination of two or more – HIV reactivates latent syphilis to reduce the immune system and leave the patient open to attack from opportunistic infections; aspects of lifestyle result in a reduced immune system which is then invaded by a host of organisms; frequent reinfection with cytomegalovirus reactivates chronic Epstein-Barr infection. These are as much supposition as the claim that HIV causes AIDS.

Having travelled through this list of micro-organisms we reach the outer edges of research where so little definitive work has been done that poorly substantiated theories abound.

To give one example: a 'new disease' which is often referred to as Chronic Fatigue Syndrome was defined in the US in the 1980s. It was dubbed 'Yuppie Flu' because it was first reported among successful, professional people in their mid-thirties. This may have been because it exclusively infected those folk or, more likely, that they were the ones with the money and confidence to insist on a medical diagnosis where other sufferers did not. The problem is characterised by fevers, sore throats, swollen lymph glands, memory loss, headaches and exhausttion. It has been described as part of a group of immunosuppressive syndromes including, but not limited to, AIDS. Now often known as myalgic encephalomyelitis, it is not known what causes it and very little work is being done to find out.

The quality of death

It is possible to become so caught up in the analysis of clinical symptoms and the microbiological zoo that one forgets that we are talking here about real human misery of the first order. These people are dying patients being cared for by suffering friends and relatives and maintained as long as possible by a straining health care system. It is important too to remember that whatever else is not known about AIDS, it is certain that this is a behavioural disease. There are things people must do, all intimate or penetrative things, before AIDS will develop. The clue to the cause of the disease is in the patient. When a leading AIDS researcher was questioned about why he never saw patients, he reportedly said: 'You don't have to live in a leper colony to cure leprosy.' It is this hubris which has led us to our current plight: research effort squandered and lives blighted by being associated with what may be a harmless passenger virus.

London psychiatrist Sidney Crown describes a representative patient struggling to come to terms with his disease;

He was a sensitive, attractive, enthusiastic music teacher. I always wanted to ask him where he bought his brightly coloured jerseys. He first came, fearful but courageous, to discuss the impact of the diagnosis on him and his partner. 'Did I really catch this from a two-week holiday in San Francisco?' he asked unbelievingly. The social stigma, not only of being suspended from his job but also of being forbidden to go to school, even after hours, to collect his books, his music, his other possessions – 'the newspapers might get hold of it' – mortified him as it did me. Over the ensuing months he talked of his apprehension about his illness, about dying, the impact on his friendship, and his attempt to occupy himself constructively by giving private music lessons. Sadly he had all the features predictive of a poor clinical outcome. Despite expert medical care and the hope occasioned by yet another 'new drug' he had to be admitted to hospital and died six months from the first diagnosis from an unresponsive chest infection. He looked pathetically physically decrepit, his face almost unrecognisable from the skin lesions of Kaposi's sarcoma.

The death of a young person is hardly likely to be uplifting. In the case of AIDS patients an already profoundly miserable experience is rendered worse by the pitiful dementia of the victims and their grotesque physical appearance, particularly considering that these were mainly young men who once took pride in their good looks.

It takes a great deal of love to stay with an AIDS patient up to the point of death. 'There are simply no words in human language to express the suffering of any one person with AIDS,' said Father Bernard Lynch who ministers to people with AIDS in New York. A clean-cut, blue-eyed athletic young man, Bernard Lynch looks more like a high-school sports teacher than a Catholic priest. He was working with the Catholic gay community in New York for three years before the AIDS epidemic even began.

Here is how he describes the death of his friend Stuart Garcia:

> You could literally see every function in his body closing down one by one. I now know that he knew we were there even when he lost consciousness, call it intuition if you will.
>
> His mom would stroke him and his sisters would stroke him and I would, and kiss his feet because the feet are so sensitive when a person dies of AIDS, the Kaposi's seems to affect the feet in an excruciating way.
>
> Eventually after a long hard struggle he expired and he looked like a bloated pig on the bed, what remained of him.

In November 1986 Dignity, an organisation of lesbian and gay Catholics, was expelled from church property in a number of dioceses including New York. In August 1987 Father Bernard Lynch was ordered by his superiors to stop his work with people with AIDS.

The immune system

AIDS has found us discussing immune suppression and T4:T8 ratios as if we know everything there is to know about the immune system. In fact it is poorly understood and many aspects of its functioning are in dispute.

It is the cellular immune system which is said to be under attack in AIDS patients though in such a complex system, a defect in one part is reflected in problems elsewhere or in compensatory efforts by other parts of the system.

One of the basic building blocks of the immune system is the white blood cell, called a lymphocyte. The cells circulate in the blood system and the lymphatic system. There are lymph nodes at points in the body – the neck, groin and armpits, for example.

A lymphocyte becomes a T cell by passing through the thymus gland (T stands for thymus). Other cells also made in the bone marrow are B lymphocytes.

To put the respective jobs of these cells very simply: when an infectious organism invades the body, it is examined and recognised by T helper cells. These cells then travel to the lymph nodes and communicate details about the invader to the B cells. B cells then produce specific antibodies – chemicals which will attack the invader alone and not other parts of the body. Natural Killer cells, another type of lymphocyte, launch in to kill cells from the body which have become infected by the outside organism.

Another T cell, called the suppressor T cell, works to calm down this activity or the powerful immune system might damage its own body in what is termed 'auto immune disease'.

It may well be that the key to AIDS lies with some other, hitherto unexplained aspect of the immune system but the relationship of some T cells to others is such an integral part of the AIDS story that it requires examination.

In order to identify cells and count them, they have to be 'tagged'. This simply means they have to be marked, in principle a concept no more complex than marking sheep with coloured dye in order to separate one part of the flock from another, which will be marked with a different colour dye.

The 'dye' in this case is a monoclonal antibody – a substance which will link on to one type of T cell and no other.

When the kits for testing T cells came on to the market, one of the first of them had a series of different monoclonal antibodies identified by numbers. Monoclonal antibody 4 reacted with T helper cells; monoclonal antibody 8 reacted with suppressor cells. They therefore came to be called T4 and T8 cells.

Once the cells are marked, they can be counted by a computer – the cells are passed in front of a laser and each one analysed in a minute fraction of a second: so many have T4 antibody, so many have T8.

In AIDS patients, researchers found early on that there were changes in the levels of T4 and T8 cells. Generally people have two helper (4) cells to one suppressor (8). AIDS patients were showing a reversal of this – they had two suppressors to one helper. This was a fascinating find and the T4:T8 ratio came to be used as a test for AIDS – reversed T4:T8 ratios meant AIDS was likely to develop in a person with fever, weight loss and so on.

Unfortunately, as usual in the AIDS story, further investigation threw up complications – healthy homosexual men also had reversed T4:T8 ratios.

As Ann Guidici Fettner writes in *The Truth About AIDS*: '[Some researchers] have speculated that the T4 cells have been so stimulated by previous and present infections as to be unable to respond anymore.' This would mean not that they weren't there but that they weren't responding to the antibodies supposed to mark them.

'One thing we don't know is why about eighty per cent of healthy gay men have 4:8 ratio reversal to some degree. Does this mean that these men are at risk for AIDS? Or do 4:8 ratios correlate with repeated infections of one kind or another? Might there be a special immune configuration among men with homosexual orientation?'

To complicate the issue further, when healthy men who were not homosexual were tested they also showed apparent peculiarities in T4:T8 ratios. Some known viral infections can cause reversals in this ratio, Cytomegalo and Epstein-Barr viruses most commonly, though other infections will also produce this condition. The difference is that in AIDS the ratios seem to stay reversed.

The reversal does not appear to affect the total number of T cells, which is often normal, the abnormality arising with an exceptional number of T suppressors. This is surprising considering another aspect of the immune systems of AIDS patients. The lowered number of helper T cells should, logically, be summoning fewer B cells to fight infection and they, correspondingly, should be producing lower detectable levels of antibodies. In fact, more antibody is being produced in AIDS patients, not less. This is of course also paradoxical in respect of the increased number of T suppressor cells relative to the T helpers. If we understand the system correctly, the T suppressors should be biologically instructing the B cells to stop producing antibody when it is not needed.

What does this mean in terms of the treatment of patients? Joe Sonnabend said:

> The ability to count T cells on a large scale came after AIDS. It was developing technology in the late nineteen-seventies and that means that what constituted a normal, healthy person's T4:T8 ratio was not known, even to this day it's probably not known. That is to say it's not known how different it is in a single person in the morning and the evening, how different between a man and a woman, how it's influenced by age, fatigue and so on. The changes in T4 and T8s in a range of diseases have yet to be established.
>
> But because there has been such attention to the T4:T8 ratios, patients have a preoccupation with their T4 cell number. They measure their progress by two or three extra or less T4 cells. However, since the measurement of T4 cells is hardly standardised between labs, it is possible for me to help a patient in a way by having his T4 cells done in a lab that I know currently produces maybe fifty per cent higher values than a prior lab. The results cannot be used in such a precise way as to measure progress.

The monoclonal antibodies were first described by Cesar Milstein in 1975; he received the Nobel Prize for this work in 1984. They were not commercially available, and therefore available for use as laboratory tools, until the late nineteen-seventies. It wasn't until the nineteen-eighties that the lasers and computers which can sort and count T cells were installed. It seems the disease arrived at the same time as equipment to analyse it became available.

An infectious disease

How infectious is AIDS? For a long time it was possible to maintain that it was not infectious at all, that it was only a behavioural disease brought about by a lifestyle which suppressed the immune system in the case of the first victims and of personal circumstances in the case of later groups to be added to the list.

Thus infections, drugs and malnutrition, sometimes in combination, damaged the immune systems of homosexuals, heroin addicts and Haitians. Haemophiliacs were immune-suppressed because of agents in their clotting factor; transfusion recipients were immune-suppressed because of drugs given as part of the medical treatment and children were immune-suppressed because their immature systems had not yet developed an effective immune system. All were therefore open to the myriad opportunistic infections which characterise AIDS.

An infectious agent was suspected because of the sudden speed of the spread of AIDS. This was not a medical fiction. Eighty-seven cases of AIDS were reported in the first six months of 1981, 365 in the corresponding period the next year and 1215 in the same period in 1983 in the US. This is not suggestive of the opportune categorisation of a disease which had been around for years. The facts do not support the suspicion that AIDS had always been with us but had not previously been diagnosed under one name until some enterprising doctors decided to write about it. The fact that kidney transplant patients suffered from cytomegalovirus and German children in the nineteen-thirties died from Pneumocystis carinii pneumonia means only that individual diseases which contributed towards the syndrome had long been known. There was a real epidemic in the US in the first part of the nineteen-eighties in some limited communities. It shocked the friends and relatives of the patients, it shocked the predominantly homosexual communities where the cases occurred, it shocked the doctors. It was not a gradual build-up of disease, it was an explosion. The fact that AIDS certainly existed a few years before it was recorded in the medical journals can only alter the story in that it sets the start date of the epidemic back a few years.

All the very early cases were, however, entirely explicable in terms of lifestyle or environment. An infectious agent was always possible and early epidemiological work like the discovery in February 1982 of the 'LA cluster' gave momentum to this theory. This work by the Centers for Disease Control found there were strong links between nine of the nineteen AIDS cases in that city. Of course, these could be behavioural links. They might all have enjoyed the same sex practices which predisposed to damage to the immune system, might all have used the same drugs, passed around the same package of pathogens in the same bathhouses. It wasn't, therefore, proof. It was good evidence.

On 16 July 1982 the CDC's Report said: 'The occurrence among the three haemophiliac cases suggests the possible transmission of an agent through blood products.'

Likewise the transfusion-related cases. Of course, there were good medical reasons why there was prior immune suppression in haemophiliacs and most transfusion patients who later developed AIDS but the evidence was piling up. In one transfusion case a woman had received contaminated blood in transfusions during a hysterectomy. She later developed weight loss, fevers, lymphadenopathy and Pneumocystis carinii pneumonia from which she died. She would not have been given drugs to knock out her immune system as transplant recipients would.

The most telling evidence for a transmissive agent is that the sexual partners of AIDS patients or people at risk for AIDS do get the disease. In the US figures for cumulative cases up to the middle of August 1988 shows 1827 apparently heterosexual people, 407 men and 1420 women, who had sexual contact with a person with AIDS or at risk for AIDS.

Even this information invites further analysis. Only one per cent of all the AIDS cases are in white people and by heterosexual transmission. Eleven per cent are black heterosexual cases and four per cent are Hispanic. These people therefore come from the poorest class of Americans, in general. One cannot tell what sort of lifestyle habits they might share with the people with whom they have sexual contact but it is unlikely that the sexual partner of a drug addict goes back to the convent at night, even given that they may not actually be intravenous drug users themselves. How many of the heterosexual contacts were women enjoying anal sex and therefore able to develop AIDS for the same reasons as homosexual men?

It is possible thus to chip away at the figures for transmission by an unknown pathogen, but a stage is reached where greater credulity is required to sustain a belief in the purely behavioural theory of the cause of AIDS than to accept that an infectious agent is involved. This is particularly true given that there have been reports of the spouses of haemophiliacs developing AIDS.

On a cautionary note: it is as well to remember in cases of AIDS, no less than any other field, that humans have an immense capacity for lies and self-deception. People are rarely called upon in the normal course of events to give full accounts of past sexual behaviour to total strangers and few can achieve it with total candour. Another factor is that serious illness distorts the patient's perception of what life was like before the illness. The AIDS patient may also be entirely dependent on a family member or a lover who would disapprove of previous behaviour, a good enough reason to play it down.

Michael Callen, a thirty-three-year-old person with AIDS, is a 'long term survivor' of the syndrome. When interviewed by Celia Farber of *Spin* magazine he had survived for six years after his diagnosis. Most of that time he had spent working in organisations for people with AIDS and agitating for better treatment for AIDS patients.

He said: 'I have gone to a great deal of trouble to find these people who claim to have had only one or two "unlucky" sexual contacts. I found ten of them in all, and each one ended up telling me they had been lying. I've known several people who were saying, in public, "I only had one or two contacts", "I only had one lover and we were monogamous", but then in the support group setting, they would regale us with tales of bathhouses and promiscuity and lovers on the side and drug use. You know, people have reasons not to stand up and say, "This is what I did". They may have families living. Maybe their lover didn't know they were playing around.'

How infectious?

The behavioural theory of AIDS and the theory that it is caused by a single pathogen are not mutually exclusive. Indeed, it is almost certainly a result of both a pathogen – or a series of them – and the prevailing lifestyle of the victim.

Gordon Stewart, Emeritus Professor of Public Health at the University of Glasgow, who worked for the World Health Organization on a survey on behavioural factors in communicable diseases, raised questions about the causation of AIDS in his report. He said to me: 'This is the behavioural disease of all behavioural diseases. Of course a germ may be at the bottom of it but it is how people behave that enables germs to cause this and many other diseases. When health damaging behaviour ceases, many diseases simply disappear and this is what should happen to AIDS. The disease comes from the co-factors and from opportunistic infections more than from HIV.'

To put it in practical terms: we do not get tuberculosis now in the Western world not because the tubercle bacillus has disappeared in the last fifty years but because of the way we live now. Legionnaire's disease may be caused by a bacteria, but it is the filthy water in which it lives and the human contact with that water which causes the disease.

A study of the epidemiology of AIDS is hopelessly confounded by repeated reference to HIV. The spirit of inquiry, scepticism and informed judgement which had guided researchers for the first three years of the epidemic simply evaporated in spring 1984 after the announcement that HIV was the cause of AIDS. All work on AIDS seemed to stop there and work on HIV was taken up; it was as if a convoy on a main highway had suddenly turned into a side road.

A look through the *Index Medicus* for 1983 shows work on patterns of risk rubbing shoulders with work on Kaposi's sarcoma, African swine fever, vesicular rosettes in the cells of affected patients and, of course, Montagnier's cautiously named lymphadenopathy-associated virus.

It also finds an editorial 'No need for panic about AIDS' which is a model of sanity. 'Even the notion that immune deficiency is acquired by means of a transmissible agent, a virus for example, is open to dispute, or at least unproven . . . mercifully the disease – whatever its causation – is neither especially infectious nor certain in its effects.'

The failure to attend to such counsels of caution led to the over-hasty identification of HIV with AIDS and therefore the association in the public mind of HIV with something approaching the bubonic plague leading to the victimisation of healthy people who were merely HIV-positive even up to the point of fire-bombing their homes.

AIDS is actually rather difficult to contract. To quote another sane human being, Arye Rubinstein, Professor of Pediatrics, Microbiology and Immunology at the Albert Einstein College of Medicine:

> When our social workers and nurses visited the homes of children with AIDS, they were impressed by the unusually close contact between family members. In many instances, children with AIDS were born to families of low socioeconomic background who lived under poor hygienic conditions. A mother and several children often lived in one room. The child with AIDS was sometimes not toilet trained and regularly shared utensils or a bed with siblings. This was not casual contact but an extremely intimate physical closeness that might be expected to facilitate transmission of disease. In spite of this, no disease was transmitted.

The 'at risk' groups develop the syndrome after transmitting large amounts of body fluids from one person to another. Small amounts seem an inefficient method.

There are few cases of health workers having developed AIDS with no apparent risk factors, despite the many cases (now running into hundreds worldwide) of 'stick injuries' – having surgical instruments, particularly syringes, penetrate the health worker's skin after being used on an AIDS patient.

It is perfectly possible that HIV is easily transmitted but AIDS is not. This proposal at least would explain the huge disparity between the numbers who are HIV antibody-positive and the people who have AIDS.

The exchange of blood products is the most efficient means of transmitting AIDS, which accounts for the transfusion-related, haemophiliac and *in utero* cases. Drug addicts also exchange blood in that they practise a method of injection known in the US as 'booting'. This involves drawing blood back into the syringe to inject again, then drawing blood back again and so on, to ensure none of the drug is wasted. Homosexuals may have semen injected into a rectum where tears in the mucosa ensure transmission directly into the bloodstream.

Whatever the cause of AIDS, or whatever co-factors may predispose a person to develop the syndrome, the means of transmission has been well established.

Are other means possible? John Seale wrote to the *Guardian* in January 1987 attacking the British government's advice, delivered to every household in the country, that there is no record of anyone becoming infected through kissing. It is worth looking at this and the ensuing letters in some detail because they encapsulate the profoundest problems of debating the AIDS case: the tendency of scientists to hush up public debate and scurry away to the pages of scientific journals; the adherence to a cherished theory regardless of the facts; the tendency to rubbish the data on which the opposing argument is based rather than rising to the challenge; the insistence that, alone among professionals, doctors should speak with one voice on public issues.

Seale cited a *Lancet* paper of December 1984 which noted the case of a sixty-one-year-old white American woman with no risk factors for AIDS. Her husband developed transfusion-related AIDS after receiving thirty units of blood products during surgery. 'The couple had not had sexual intercourse for three years, since the patient was rendered impotent by the operation that repaired his abdominal aorta, but had had exchange of saliva by kissing during that time.' The woman had HIV itself (though not, interestingly enough, antibodies to it).

Seale went on to note a paper in *Science* where researchers detected HIV in the saliva of eight out of eighteen people who had antibodies to the virus.

This is, of course, a debate about the infectivity of the virus and no one was purporting to prove by this that the virus causes AIDS. The theory that HIV causes AIDS had been accepted without close examination for almost three years by this time.

Sir Donald Acheson, the government's chief medical officer, replied:

On the basis of current epidemiological evidence, it is clear that the HIV virus is passed on either as a result of penetrative sexual intercourse or the injection of blood and blood products or by transmission of infection from mother to baby before or during birth.

Although virus particles have been found in saliva, there is no evidence that it has transmitted infection. . . . I can therefore reassure your readers that there is no sound evidence that the AIDS virus has been transmitted by kissing. . . . The scientific arguments justifying this view will be dealt with in more detail in a letter to the *British Medical Journal*.

Why he wished to continue the debate in another publication is a matter for conjecture. It was not because the matters involved are too complex for *Guardian* readers. The letter in the *British Medical Journal* was no more complex than the *Guardian* letters already published. Perhaps some *Guardian* readers would not have understood the debate but, after all, the *Guardian* is full of items which not every reader will understand. How many readers of the education pages understand the financial pages and vice versa?

Before the *BMJ* letter was published, another person wrote to the *Guardian* noting a report in the *Lancet* of September 1986 about a boy who had HIV from a blood transfusion who bit his brother and infected him with the virus. 'Sir Donald is, perhaps, paying too little regard to virology studies and too much to epidemiological evidence which is inadequate and incomplete,' wrote Christopher Monckton. 'Sir Donald and his team would do well not to pooh-pooh such currently unusual routes of transmission as saliva. They should, instead, study the influence of environmental, bacterial and viral co-factors which may, if left undetected, cause AIDS to spread in unexpected ways and with surprising speed.'

Sir Donald passed the task of replying, in the *British Medical Journal*, to Joseph Smith, one of those civil servants who were now found to be commenting on such matters as:

> Some forms of open mouthed kissing can be associated with considerable transfer of saliva. In epidemiological studies intimate kissing is confounded with sexual intercourse, which makes it difficult to be sure of the precise role of each in the transmission of infection. . . . there is also indirect evidence from the relative safety of oral sex. Though semen can transmit infection when deposited in the rectum or vagina, the evidence suggests that it is probably not associated with risk by the oral route.
>
> There is, moreover, no evidence of salivary transmission to health care workers such as dentists and it has been suggested that there is an inhibitory factor for HIV present in saliva.

On the two case reports cited he comments that the papers which report relatively easy transmission of HIV are in error. Of the sixty-one-year-old woman he noted: 'Inadequate detail was given of the type and frequency of contacts between the woman and her impotent husband or of any other sexual contacts. Though it was assumed that her husband became infected through a transfusion during the surgical operation that rendered him impotent, no information is given in the paper about the infectivity of the blood donors concerned. A single case report with incomplete information is an insufficient basis for the argument that kissing has resulted in the transmission of HIV.'

On the case of the mordacious child Smith writes: 'The method of transmission between the two boys was unknown, although it was speculated that saliva in a bite on the forearm might have been responsible. Inoculation of infected material is recognised as a method of transmission of HIV; this case is thus not directly relevant to the dangers or safety of kissing.'

But aren't we here talking about the inoculation of saliva? If HIV isn't in saliva in any quantity, how can it be inoculated into someone in a fraternal bite? And how was it passed on from the African green monkey in a bite, for those who favour that theory?

Smith's criticism of the limitations of the papers looks a little thin when he quotes, in the same letter, from two papers he marshals to demonstrate that there is HIV in the semen of infected people – another matter about which Dr John Seale is in doubt.

Dr Smith quotes papers by Ho and Zagury, the former of whom found HIV in the semen of a healthy homosexual and the second cultured HIV from the semen of two AIDS patients.

Whenever supporters of the HIV theory want to prove there is HIV in semen, these two papers are always quoted. The two papers cover the heroic efforts employed by researchers to recover virus from the semen of three people. After twelve days using a variety of methods, the HIV was recovered but the same type of techniques are necessary to culture it from saliva or tears. Why is semen considered a more potent transmissible fluid than saliva? Presumably because this fits in with the theory that HIV causes AIDS and if it is accepted that one is as likely to be infected by saliva as semen, that considerably weakens the case for HIV.

Another issue which emerged from this exchange of letters was the toothbrush story. Those *Guardian* readers, too plebeian to comprehend the scientific arguments, nevertheless had some interesting points to make. One reminded Sir Donald that all of the UK's 23 million households were given a leaflet which gave them advice on how not to 'die of ignorance'. The leaflet explicitly forbade sharing the toothbrush of someone who was infected. Why was this if there is no danger in saliva?

Roderic Griffiths from the Central Birmingham Health Authority gives an answer when responding to an attack on his advice that sharing toothbrushes cannot transmit AIDS:

We advise callers that slack hygiene is unwise; that hepatitis B may well be transmitted by such practices as sharing a toothbrush; but that to avoid AIDS, the most important thing for all of us to think about is our sexual behaviour.

To frighten people with one-in-a-million risks is pointless. It distracts people from the real issue of convincing people that it is who they have sex with, not which toothbrush they use, which will affect their chance of getting AIDS.

The use of another person's toothbrush seems to be a particularly ghastly item in the inventory of human congress anyway, and should be stopped, AIDS or no AIDS.

What the kissing and toothbrush stories tell us is how uncertain everything is. No one really knows whether saliva or the amount of foreign blood one might brush into the gums on a toothbrush or semen ejaculated into a mouth which may have gingivitis are a realistic mode of transmission of AIDS.

One can sympathise with Sir John Rawlins' comment, also in the *BMJ*: 'It seems that the only safe course is to limit sexual congress to manual fondling, which suggests a bleak future for the human species.'

All the best authorities can do is to try hard to prioritise the risks and present them to the public in a way which will avoid panic. Every medical paper which presents an epidemiological fact related to single cases can be challenged by another. There is only safety in numbers.

Consider the case of the lesbians. It has long been asked why, if AIDS is God's punishment for homosexual sin, has He seen fit to place lesbians in the very lowest risk category? Is there a concealed spiritual message in this? Unfortunately, as usual, a case has been reported which ruins a good line.

Lesbians

A *Lancet* letter of July reports on female-to-female transmission of HIV in a twenty-four-year-old unmarried dancer from the Philippines. She travelled and worked as a dancer in Mediterranean countries from 1981 to 1983. 'She had encounters with many women of different nationalities. Orogenital contact was practised. In 1983 she returned to the Philippines where she re-established a steady relationship with her previous partner. She denied all heterosexual contact and intravenous drug abuse, and she had no history of blood transfusion.'

A San Francisco AIDS Foundation leaflet, *Lesbians and AIDS*, suggests that at least some lesbians are at risk from their sexual practices:

Unsafe Sex Practices for Lesbians at Risk
Unprotected cunnilingus (especially during menstruation)

Unprotected hand/finger-to-vagina or anus contact, especially if you
   have cuts on your hands
Sharing needles (IV needles, skin-piercing needles)
Blood contact of any kind, including menstrual blood and sharing
   IV needles
Urine or faeces in mouth or vagina
Unprotected rimming (anal-oral contact)
Fisting (hand in rectum/vagina)
Sharing sex toys that have contact with body fluids.

Regardless of the fact that some lesbians must do each of these things,
or other lesbians would not warn against them, it is the case that
lesbians seem to be at extremely low risk. It is therefore worth noting,
merely for the sake of the recognition of human charity on its rare
appearances, that lesbians have been among the most compassionate
and giving of supporters for people with AIDS in San Francisco and
other centres of the epidemic. A great deal of the help and comfort
which men dying from AIDS need has come from lesbian volunteers
despite their own virtual immunity. Of course, a self-righteous attack
on male homosexuals by the majority population would certainly also
affect lesbians.

Women to men

Female-to-male transmission of AIDS is rare, though it has been
demonstrated as well as any other aspect of epidemiology in the
progress of this disease. The report quoted most often, perhaps because
it is so clear, refers to one woman and two men.

A thirty-seven-year-old bisexual man who lived in Cleveland, Ohio,
travelled frequently between New York and Cleveland from 1981 to
1983. He was an active homosexual and New York was the best place
in the world to be homosexually active on a weekend business trip. In
1983 he developed the familiar pattern of sickness culminating in
Pneumocystis carinii pneumonia and death.

His thirty-three-year-old wife, who had been married to him for ten
years, had no other sexual partners and no intravenous drug use. 'She
had had vaginal intercourse with her husband twice monthly, accompanied by heavy mouth kissing but no other form of sexual contact.'
Nevertheless, eighteen months after her husband, she too developed
Pneumocystis carinii pneumonia and died.

The twenty-six-year-old next-door neighbour of that busy Cleveland
home started a sexual relationship with the woman several months after
her husband's death. 'They began to cohabit and participated for

approximately a year in daily vaginal intercourse accompanied by heavy mouth kissing . . . he reported no other form of sexual contact with the woman and no history of homosexuality, drug abuse or contact with prostitutes,' but he too went down with generalised lymphadenopathy and oral thrush. The Cleveland doctors reporting the case noted that it showed that 'frequent but traditional sexual practices' had their dangers.

Having sex with a promiscuous homosexual or bisexual man is clearly an activity well up on the league table of AIDS risks. In general, AIDS is not easy to acquire and much of the hysteria generated about it, particularly in the US, has derived from a prudish reluctance to talk in public about perfectly commonplace human phenomena – vaginal, oral and anal sex. As Surgeon General C. Everett Koop said: 'Many people, especially our youth, are not receiving information that is vital to their future health and wellbeing because of our reticence in dealing with the subjects of sex, sexual practices and homosexuality . . . the silence must end.'

He has a long way to go in that battle – the San Francisco AIDS Foundation was forbidden to send out information on safe sex practices, safe sex videos and other material through the mail because it was considered pornographic.

Three

Virus Hunters

The cancer viruses

IT HAD LONG been observed that in a flock of chickens if one had cancer, many would get it – unmistakable swollen tumours and a wasting away of the animal. Obviously this was of some interest to poultry farmers and to people who kept a few chickens in the back yard. But cancer scientists took an interest in this humble fowl disease. Why should so many get the cancer? Was it something in their feed? Something in the air? Were they passing it on like an infectious disease? This was a problem: conventional wisdom says cancer is not infectious.

The tumour itself, if transplanted, would cause the same tumour in the recipient. Peyton Rous at the Rockefeller Institute for Medical Research examined this phenomenon in 1910. Filters were commonly used to separate bacteria – at that time the smallest known infectious agents – from the matter they were infecting. Rous pulverised a tumour, filtered it and tested the 'filtrate' on tumour-free animals. It caused a tumour in the new fowl. There was an infectious agent in the filtrate which caused cancer.

This was a major breakthrough in medical research. It shared the distinction with other great breakthroughs in medicine of being ignored at the time. As Renato Dulbecco writes in his memoir on Peyton Rous: 'For about forty years this momentous discovery had little impact, because the minds of scientists were not prepared to think of viruses as agents of cancer. It was expedient to say that the chicken tumour was not a cancer, but some kind of reaction to the virus more akin to inflammation than neoplasia, and perhaps a peculiarity of chicken biology. Peyton Rous soon recognised himself that the tumour would not be accepted as a cancer *because* it was a cell-free extract,' (i.e. only something smaller than cells would penetrate the filter).

This reaction is interesting in the light of the behaviour of scientists on the establishment side of the AIDS industry when their position is challenged by new data: first, restate accepted rules as if they are fact; second, question your opponent's powers of observation and, by implication, scientific skill; third, concede that there may be an exception in this case but it is peculiar and in no way contradicts the general rule. Attacks on the establishment position, however, are welcomed with an extension of theory which is restated to such an extent that it is difficult to extricate the facts from the theorising.

Rous identified another two chicken viruses in the following years until lack of recognition, and the demands of the First World War made him leave this work. During the war he developed a solution for suspending the red cells of blood so they could be used for transfusion. This is still in use and is known as the Rous–Turner solution.

The turning point was the independent discovery in 1933 by Richard Shope of a tumour of cottontail rabbits which seemed to be transmitted by a virus. Rous returned to studying tumours in animals, his open mind leaving him increasingly uncertain about the role of viruses in cancer over the next three decades. Viruses seemed to be changing, to be showing variation – sometimes they produced tumours, sometimes they did not. Rous' guiding principle, as a model of good sense, is worth repeating: 'How far should one be led by the assumption that certain tumours may be due to viruses? Only so far as to make tests with these growths. The tumour problem has withstood the most corrosive reasoning. Yet since what one thinks determines what one does in cancer research, as in all else, it is as well to think something. And it may prove worthwhile to think that one or more tumours of unknown causes are due to viruses.'

The theory was a tool of thought, not a master of it.

Rous was awarded the Nobel Prize for his work in 1966. He was eighty-seven and was to die four years later. It had been fifty-six years since he made the discovery which earned him the prize.

That there were infectious diseases was not news. Chinese accounts of the tenth century BC report a disease which is almost certainly smallpox. Vaccination against the smallpox virus was known at least from the eighteenth century AD. It was not known what this infectious agent was until the bacteriologists Frederick Twort and Felix Herelle, in 1915 and 1917 respectively, identified viruses within bacteria. They demonstrated that viruses were separate particles much tinier than bacteria. It is now known in fact that there are some viruses almost as large as bacteria and some bacteria as small as viruses. Identification and classification of viruses has continued through this century. Because their small size was shared with some bacteria this could not be used as the distinguishing feature of them. It was thought that their inability to replicate outside a cell they were infecting could be used as a distinguishing characteristic but this too is shared with some bacteria which more commonly are complete organisms. Now viruses are characterised by their simple organisation and their means of replication: a virus is a bundle of genetic material wrapped in a protein coat. It does not contain sufficient mechanism for its own replication but must enter a cell in a host – and there are plant as well as animal viruses – in order to use part of the mechanism of the cell to reproduce itself.

Cancer research

The direction which AIDS research took is so deeply rooted in the history of cancer research in the second half of this century that it is necessary to know a little about cancer before it is possible to understand why cancer laboratories and cancer researchers took such a leading role in research into AIDS.

Knowing about chicken cancers is all very well, but common sense indicates cancer in both humans and animals relates to the division of body cells, the way they reproduce themselves. At some stage in life, almost always in later life, an organ begins to overproduce cells which invade the surrounding tissues. Often this is followed by a spread to other sites in the body by way of the circulatory systems: referred to as metastasis. Of the one hundred different forms of human cancer, each have their own age of onset, rate of growth and tendency to spread. Cancer is not reversible though it can sometimes be attacked with radiation or surgery, both of which will destroy a tumour, or far less successfully with drug treatment (chemotherapy). Very occasionally, spontaneous remission does occur and a patient recovers.

There seems to be a programme to turn on cancer at a particular age in particular people but what is it that turns the disease on? Environmental factors certainly have some effect: workers in the leather industries suffer from bladder cancer because of the chemicals they use at work; smokers suffer more lung cancer than non-smokers. Apart from this small percentage of environmentally induced cancers – and cancer is by no means inevitable, even in these circumstances – the reason why a cancer starts at a particular time in a particular individual is still a mystery.

Perhaps one of the genes of a particular organ starts to go wrong on its own and begins to overproduce. Perhaps a virus gets into a cell and converts or 'transforms' the genes into enemies.

Many viruses were found in animal and human tumours by scientists pursuing these theories. Most of them did not cause cancer. About twenty types of animal virus did cause cancer but they were all a very special type of virus: the *oncogenic retrovirus*.

Oncogenic viruses are those which give rise to tumours – oncology is the study of tumours. Retroviruses are a particular class of virus whose name comes from their genetic programme.

The genetic code – the information which instructs each cell in how to reproduce itself – is contained in DNA (deoxyribonucleic acid). DNA is present in all body cells of all species including unicellular organisms and viruses.

In this model it is best to see DNA as the 'double helix' – two corkscrews wrapped around each other – of coded information as first described by Francis Crick and James Watson in 1953, for which they received the Nobel Prize in 1962. RNA, for this purpose, is best seen as short strands of information, smaller segments of the information for which DNA encodes the entire sequence.

The genetic code of a retrovirus is RNA (ribonucleic acid) which is transcribed ('rewritten as') DNA by an enzyme called reverse transcriptase. Once the DNA is present in the cell it locks itself into the cell's own DNA. The picture is finally presented of a virus entirely dependent on the cell's genetic material – it can replicate only when the cell itself replicates.

This is a complex subject but it is integral to the AIDS story, so I will attempt a model which should, it is hoped, do no great damage to the truth. Imagine a word processor which prints those business letters which find themselves in so many wastepaper baskets – the kind which are full of clichés, stock phrases and jargon words. All those exist in the machine but they are not connected. The word processor has a series of words already made up but they are not in sentences. These stand for RNA. Words are the same as sentences, of course, sentences are just arrangements of words in an ordered sequence. The computer programme which commands the writing of the business letter is the reverse transcriptase, it transcribes RNA into DNA – transcribes words into sentences. Once this letter has been constructed, it can be reproduced as often as required but however often it is photocopied, the words and phrases will not become random again, they are locked into their order.

The retrovirus, then, is locked into a cell. It cannot reproduce without using the cell's own reproductive mechanism. Back to the chickens.

Peyton Rous's chicken tumour was caused by one such retrovirus, the Rous sarcoma virus. When the cell reproduces, along with the retrovirus, it overproduces. It may then cause a tumour, a massive overproliferation of cells. This is possible because the Rous sarcoma virus has an extra piece of information – an oncogene. Without this, the retrovirus would live in peace with its host until the host died of natural causes. This is the clue to the mystery of those viruses which cause tumours and those which do not: if they do not have the 'transforming' gene which will turn a peaceful into an aggressive virus, there will be no tumour.

The entire field is very new. Reverse transcriptase was discovered only in 1970 by Howard Temin and David Baltimore, who received the Nobel Prize for this work in 1975.

Oncogenes were discovered in 1970 by Peter Duesberg and Peter Vogt. They had long been believed to exist, but believing and proving are different things. Duesberg and Vogt defined in molecular and genetic terms the first 'transforming' gene which caused a tumour.

Could these steps be proof of the gathering momentum towards ascribing causes to the cancers, leading to cures for them?

The cancer research programme now received its greatest stimulus. On 22 January 1971, in his State of the Union address, President Richard Nixon declared war on cancer. He said: 'I will ask for an appropriation of an extra one hundred million dollars to launch an intensive campaign to find a cure for cancer and I will ask later for whatever additional funds can be effectively used. The time has come in America where the same kind of concentrated effort that split the atom and took man to the moon should be turned to conquering this dread disease.'

As will have been realised from other excursions of Richard Nixon, the word hubris was not one which made frequent appearances in his vocabulary. This speech, which heralded the Cancer Act and other efforts by governments and charities worldwide, meant more money and resources were spent on cancer than on any other disease before or since. The field was awash with money. It was the time of hope and riches before the oil crisis, the research institutes were buoyant, the manufacturers who supplied them with equipment had full order books, a footnote in the annals of cancer research was a passport to a doctorate, the Nobel Prize glowed in the distance like the sun.

The cancer research programme was far from being an overwhelming success. By the mid-nineteen-eighties articles were beginning to appear in major journals such as 'Progress Against Cancer?' in the *New England Journal of Medicine*. Here authors looked dispassionately at the figures and noted that the cancer mortality rate continued to rise slowly from the nineteen-fifties to the nineteen-eighties despite the vast research effort. Moreover, there was no breakthrough just around the corner. The authors bitterly remarked: 'We are losing the war against cancer, notwithstanding progress against several uncommon forms of the disease, improvements in palliation, and extension of the productive years of life. A shift in research emphasis, from research on treatment to research on prevention, seems necessary if substantial progress against cancer is to be forthcoming.'

One of the theories on which fortune smiled was the theory that viruses caused cancer. It had a head start on other theories, because of earlier work in the field, and it promised great things. Consequently some great minds went into the virus cancer research programme. At one time, viruses were being found in almost every tumour, particularly retroviruses. Peter Duesberg, Professor of Molecular Biology at Berkeley, was part of the virus cancer research programme. He said:

> We know that mice and chickens contain fifty to a hundred retroviruses which never cause disease. Viruses seemed to be at least a plausible cause of human cancer, based on animal work, and that programme has produced a lot of good things for science but has not identified the cause of human cancer.
>
> When you're in the retrovirus business you can detect a retrovirus. When you look at a disease, you can look for the retrovirus. We have done that before with multiple sclerosis, we have done it with leukaemias, we have done it with sarcomas, and in almost all cases a virus was found sooner or later.
>
> What was not emphasised by many of these laboratories was that the same viruses were subsequently always found in healthy carriers and that's why the virus cancer programme is essentially a failure.

Most connections between cancer and viruses are mere association: hepatitis B virus is associated with a high rate of cancer of the liver many years after first infection. There may well be an infectious agent in cancer of the cervix and cancer of the penis because a person with one of these is likely to have a sexual partner at a higher risk than average of developing the other.

It is possible that a virus challenges a human organ repeatedly, damaging the liver or the cervix in frequent tiny attacks. This means the cells of the organ have to replenish themselves faster than they would in the natural course of events. The greater the number of cells replicating, the higher the chance that one will 'go wrong' and start replicating out of control – a cancer. If every hepatitis B infection caused liver cancer, or if every liver cancer was in a person with hepatitis B, it would all be so much easier. It was not to be so; the viruses contribute to the risk of a cancer developing, they do not cause cancers.

Robert Gallo and the human retroviruses

The only other success story of the virus cancer programme was the announcement of the isolation of the first human retrovirus – human T-cell leukaemia virus, by Robert Gallo, Chief of the Laboratory of Tumor Cell Biology at the National Cancer Institute, Maryland, USA.

Robert Gallo is seen as the hero and the villain of the AIDS story. He has been described as 'champion of the single cause theory' meaning he believes AIDS is caused by a single agent with no co-factors. He is quoted as saying: 'Who needs co-factors when you've been hit by a truck?' He pursues his theory with a vigour which is impressive even to those who do not like him. He is a skilful communicator, popular with the media and in particular the medical and scientific correspondents who are invited into his confidence; general reporters develop an immunity to charm.

Gallo was born in Connecticut in 1937. Much is made of the incident when, at the age of thirteen, he saw his sister dying of leukaemia. He took a medical degree and began as soon as he could to study leukaemia in the laboratory – his nature was too restless to allow him to enjoy work with patients. Within two years of finishing his degree he was working at the National Cancer Institute where he was to stay for more than twenty-five years.

The young Gallo was immediately interested in the virus-cancer programme, showing most enthusiasm for the theory that viruses came from outside the body to infect and cause a cancer by some as yet unknown mechanism. There was another theory of endogenous (passenger) viruses which might cause disease in the presence of carcinogenic (cancer-causing) agents, but this theory has fallen into disfavour. Gallo backed the right horse and became deeply involved in the subject of RNA viruses immediately after Temin and Baltimore discovered reverse transcriptase.

Gallo describes his own thought processes: 'In 1970, when Temin and Baltimore came on reverse transcriptase, I was studying DNA polymerases in blood cells. DNA polymerases are enzymes that assemble DNA; reverse transcriptase is a member of this group, albeit an unusual one. Under the influence of Temin's ideas I decided to search for reverse transcriptase in human leukaemic cells, hoping to find a retrovirus there.'

Seek and ye shall find. But it was necessary to use the correct techniques. The electron microscope, which could detect objects thousands of times smaller than those available to an optic microscope, was 'a cumbersome tool for the purpose' according to Gallo. Moreover, human leukaemic cells had been studied under electron microscopes and no virus particles had been identified.

Gallo and co-workers laboured to refine the test for reverse transcriptase until the enzymes could be detected in leukaemic cells. They did find what seemed to be reverse transcriptase but in such small amounts that it could easily have been some other substance mimicking the behaviour of the key enzyme. They needed a much larger supply of the cells with this questionable virus.

This was where Gallo's real skill, and that of his colleagues, came into play. In years to come he will be known as a first-class bench scientist who made significant contributions to the development of cell lines in which viruses could be studied. A plant protein, phytohemagglutinin, had been discovered in the nineteen-sixties. It would induce white blood cells to grow in tissue culture. Gallo's lab noticed that after such stimulation, some T cells released a growth factor. They would culture T cells to harvest this growth factor and would use it to stimulate T cells which were growing with phytohemagglutinin. Gallo now had T cell lines growing and rapidly reproducing – a perfect set-up for any experiment he chose to perform with them.

There was something of a diversion on the path to find the cause of human leukaemia. In 1975 Robert Gallo published a paper saying he had isolated a new human virus – human leukaemia virus 23.

Gallo was jubilant, it was the justification for years of dedication. 'We got permanently growing cell lines eventually, and it was a great eureka. We succeeded ten times in ten different cell lines, and we thought we had made the discovery, the genuine article, that retroviruses exist in humans. A year or more of analysis went by. We thought it was a triumph.'

This period of research turned from being Gallo's greatest triumph to date into his greatest disaster. When other scientists looked at this virus they discovered it was a mixture of three animal viruses: from a gibbon, a baboon and a woolly monkey.

The term for this is contamination – the human serum from a leukaemia patient had been contaminated by animal viruses. The way this can occur is well-known and laboratories go to great lengths to avoid it. Viruses are worked on in 'hoods' which are basically lab benches surrounded by a clear plastic shield in which a fan takes air, which may contain particles of viruses or other material, out of the lab. It is always possible for scientists to bring in contaminants from outside, despite the measures taken to avoid this, or for lab equipment used in the hoods to be contaminated or for material in other hoods in the same room to pass over and contaminate new material. One contamination is probable in a long research period, two is possible, three is unlikely.

As Gallo said: 'I was depressed, dumbfounded, angry. It was the low point of my whole career. It was almost the last nail in the coffin of the field of retrovirology. The programme died, and all the good that came out of it, like interleukin-2, which would be so important in fighting cancers, didn't seem to matter, to me or to the world. I became more cynical, tougher, less happy. I mean, what could it be but sabotage? One contamination can occur, but three? In fifteen years I had had one contamination from a mouse. But three?'

Robin Weiss, another leading cancer researcher who is now working in the field of AIDS, played a leading role in determining the non-human component of human leukaemia 23. He said: 'In the late seventies everyone was laughing at Gallo, they'd say: "There goes Gallo again discovering another human retrovirus." When he went to scientific meetings people would laugh at him. Every fashionable lab was going into oncogenes. He said man can't be the exception, man must be able to be infected with retroviruses too. He proved us wrong, he found a retrovirus which causes leukaemia.'

A leukaemia breakthrough?

The connection between AIDS and leukaemia is almost nil. There is a slight connection in that Robert Gallo and those who followed his line of reasoning connected the two for reasons which will be demonstrated. In order to render this accessible, it is worth a quick aside to define leukaemia: it is a malignant disease of the blood-forming organs marked by a proliferation of leukocytes (white cells which include all kinds of T cells among their number) and a reduced number of red cells. Leukaemia is classified according to three facts: first the character and duration of the disease; second the type of cell involved; and third the increase or non-increase in the number of abnormal cells – in effect it can be either leukaemic or aleukaemic.

Acute lymphoid leukaemia is, therefore, a disease whose onset is fast, which involves lymphocytes and is characterised by a massive increase in abnormal cells in the blood. Heredity is involved in some leukaemias and radiation is certainly a factor in myelocytic leukaemia – the higher the dose, the more likely it is to develop. Acute leukaemia will cause a tendency to bleed, joint pains, enlargement of lymph nodes, liver and spleen and an increased susceptibility to infection.

Robert Gallo and his colleagues took cells from leukaemic patients, grew them with phytohemagglutinin and interleukin-2 and managed to produce reverse transcriptase. They had found a retrovirus. They called it HTLV-I: Human T-cell Leukaemia Virus I.

They now needed to find the disease which it caused. The patients from whom the virus had been isolated had a cancer of the T4 cells accompanied by skin abnormalities. This was a well described condition (mycosis fungoides or Sézary T-cell leukaemia) and only a small fraction of patients with it had HTLV-I. The quest for the disease led to Japan where in 1977 Kiyoshi Takatsuki of Kyoto University described something he called Adult T-cell Leukaemia which killed within a few months of diagnosis and was characterised by an explosive proliferation of leukaemic cells. It was heavily concentrated in Kyushu and

Shikoku, Japan's southernmost islands. Gallo remarked: 'Such cluster-ing suggested the disease might be caused by an infectious agent.'

It was clear the Japanese were well on the way to describing the virus also. Yorio Hinuma of Kyoto University and Isao Miyoshi of Kochi University had grown a line of cells from leukaemic patients which were releasing retrovirus particles. In a curious dress rehearsal for the AIDS story Gallo and his team had an isolate from a patient which Hinuma and his team also seemed to have. Gallo notes: 'All available data indicated that the virus coming from Miyoshi's cells was identical with HTLV-I.'

Gallo claims he and his colleagues isolated the first examples of HTLV-I in 1978–9 and that the results were published in 1980 and early 1981. To delay publication for up to three years is uncharacteristic in a man not given to false modesty.

Gallo is credited with isolating and describing the first human retrovirus. Japanese and American researchers confirmed by analysing the RNA of both isolates that the Japanese and American viruses were related strains of the same virus. They could never be exactly the same because of the mutations which occur as the virus replicates, but the RNA sequence was close enough in the two isolates.

Once the virus had been described, other laboratories looked for it. It was found in black patients born in the US, Caribbean countries or South America; Caribbean-born black people in England, Africans and Japanese. 'What could tie these disparate regions together?' mused Gallo.

The answer he came up with was the slave trade. Miyoshi in Japan found Japanese macaques had antibodies to HTLV-I and he suggested the monkeys had the disease first and infected people. Researchers at Göttingen, Germany, and in Gallo's lab found that many species of African monkeys had antibodies which reacted with HTLV-I. African green monkey and chimpanzee viruses were most closely related to the virus Gallo had found in leukaemic cells.

Gallo suggested:

HTLV-I originated in Africa where it infected many species of Old World primates, including human beings. It reached the Americas along with the slave trade.

Curiously, it may well have arrived in Japan the same way. In the sixteenth century Portuguese traders travelled to Japan and stayed specifically in the islands where HTLV-I is now endemic. Along with them they brought both African slaves and monkeys, as contem-porary Japanese works of art show, and either one or the other may have carried the virus.

The discovery of HTLV-I infection on Hokkaido, one of the northern islands of Japan, immediately challenged this view of events but Gallo and his colleagues have remained attached to the monkey-virus theory.

So, why is it thought that this virus causes the leukaemia? First because of the coincidence between virus and leukaemia – find one and you will find the other, Gallo says. Moreover, infected infants born in the endemic area of southern Japan have the same chance of developing adult T-cell leukaemia whether they stay there or move to another part of the world.

In presenting this as an argument that his virus does cause this leukaemia, Gallo is, in the opinion of some, going beyond the evidence. The fact that some children will invariably get adult T-cell leukaemia in time, regardless of whether they are near to or thousands of miles from the supposed centre of HTLV-I infection, argues against an infectious agent and for a genetic cause.

Gallo further notes that there is a difference in the arrangement of infection between T cells infected in the laboratory and T cells infected in a patient. In the lab culture, the virus infects different parts of the cell at random. In a given patient, the virus is always seen to infect the same chromosome in every cell. This implies the cells are all clones of the same original infected cell. 'It also implies,' says Gallo, 'that the infection preceded the origin of the tumour, because if the virus had entered the cells of an existing multicellular tumour, the viral sequences would be found in a different place in each cell of the tumour.'

'So,' says Peter Duesberg, 'you have a virus which infects many T cells. If one of the millions or billions of T cells infected becomes the clonal precursor of a T-cell leukaemia, many years later, we have no evidence that the virus caused the leukaemic transformation. In fact we have millions or billions of "control cells" in the same patient to show that it didn't.'

Duesberg's criticisms of the claims for a direct relationship between HTLV-I and T-cell leukaemia mirror his criticisms of the claims that AIDS is caused by HIV. The most obvious question is why don't people with HTLV-I develop leukaemia? There are simply too many people infected with the virus but perfectly healthy for the virus to be the cause.

The incidence of adult T-cell leukaemia in Japan, Duesberg points out, is estimated to be only 0.06 per cent based on 339 cases of T-cell leukaemia among 600,000 subjects who are antibody-positive for HTLV-I. Why is this?

Because of the latency period, responds Gallo. It will cause leukaemia, but it may take as long as forty years.

So, when will we see a controlled trial to prove your theory? asks Duesberg.

The point is that when the time from infection to the appearance of the disease is so flexible – earlier estimates put it at five years – a great deal is being left to chance. Robert Gallo would be long dead before a controlled cohort study of HTLV-I carriers could show whether his theory is correct or not.

HTLV-I needs all its genetic material for its own replication, Duesberg notes, and if it isn't causing cancer as soon as it gets into a cell but is peacefully replicating along with the cell, where does the characteristic for starting a leukaemia come from?

In the nineteen-seventies Duesberg defined the genetic nature of retroviruses and produced a 'genetic map' which is true of all retroviruses. There are three genes, *gag*, *pol* and *env* and a series of repetitive sequences called 'long terminal repeats' which need not concern us here.

The *gag* encodes the protein core which encloses the virus's RNA and reverse transcriptase molecules; the *pol* gene encodes the reverse transcriptase and the *env* encodes the protein 'envelope' in which it is all wrapped. In addition to this, Gallo's lab discovered another gene in HTLV-I, a so-called *tat* gene.

Could this not be performing the 'transforming' function: transforming a cell the virus has entered into a cancerous cell? No, says Duesberg, unless it happens every time.

If it was a transforming gene, every infected cell should be transformed. That is clearly not the case, there are millions of carriers of that virus who do not have leukaemia. The percentage of carriers who get leukaemia is not significantly higher than the percentage of spontaneous leukaemias in virus-free people.

In cells infected with this retrovirus, transformation is an incredibly rare event and the virus has nothing to do with it. By comparison Rous sarcoma virus transforms every infected cell. That is the difference between a retrovirus which causes a disease and one which does not.

In addition he says the *tat* gene must be essential for viral replication: if the gene is removed by a technique called 'deletion analysis', the virus does not grow any more, it therefore cannot be a gene which performs a rare, non-essential function like causing a leukaemia in the host.

Even those who do believe HTLV-I is a cause of leukaemia in some people are at a loss to understand why leukaemia is caused in fewer than one in a hundred carriers. Clearly there is some other factor working as well as the HTLV-I, or perhaps HTLV-I plays no role in the cause of leukaemia at all.

Ironically, as Gallo and his team ploughed on with their T-cell virus, two other researchers started looking at interleukin-2 which Gallo's lab had developed only as a tool for growing T-cell lines. Kendall A. Smith at the Dartmouth Medical School and Hans Wigzell of the Karolinska Institute in Stockholm investigated how interleukin-2 and its precursor interleukin-1 function as part of the immune system. In doing so they made a genuine contribution to the understanding of human health and sickness. A greater understanding of the immune system as it functions efficiently has been one of the more pressing medical needs of the past decade.

In another mirror of the AIDS story, HTLV-I now began to be connected with a range of other illnesses in addition to human T-cell leukaemia. The problem of the widespread infection with HTLV-I with no clinical disease was solved by Max Essex suggesting that: 'People infected with the virus are prone to other infections, perhaps because some infected T cells, although not transformed, are functionally impaired.'

It was suggested that such 'impaired' T cells may contribute to leukaemias of the B cells and that HTLV-I is associated with a neurological disease resembling multiple sclerosis. As Robert Gallo writes: 'It seems clear that the overall impact of HTLV-I on public health is just beginning to be realised' (1987). Put another way: viruses are where you look for them and they will be found in people with a range of diseases. They will also be found in healthy individuals. In a manner which also foreshadows developments in the HIV story, variants of this virus were described and diseases began to be ascribed to them. HTLV-II was discovered in 1982 by Gallo's group in collaboration with researchers at the University of California School of Medicine at Los Angeles. It was found in a young white man suffering from hairy-cell leukaemia and subsequently claimed to be the cause of this rare form of leukaemia, though Gallo himself has been somewhat cautious in his own pronouncements about the pathogenicity of HTLV-II.

Whether or not the two HTL viruses are responsible for leukaemias, their discovery was a remarkable laboratory tour de force. Within a decade of the discovery of reverse transcriptase which allowed retroviruses to be identified, the first human retrovirus had been discovered. As Gallo himself notes, there were two preconditions for its discovery: 'The first, a sensitive assay for the virus, was provided by the discovery of reverse transcriptase. The second was the establishment of a method for growing T cells in the laboratory.'

Given the appropriate equipment, any laboratory worker could now duplicate this procedure and retroviruses could be added to all the other viruses which could be obtained from human tissue. John Beldekas has done as much bench work of this type as any other researcher. He commented: 'As a researcher growing a virus, I could take a cell from your body and under the appropriate laboratory conditions I could coax out a lot of viruses that you have been exposed to. That doesn't mean you are a walking carrier that's shedding viruses and it doesn't mean you are potentially infectious. The carrying of these organisms we have been exposed to is called persistence – they persist within us and we can find them if we look with the right techniques.'

However impressive this lab work was, it was a poor return on the investment of billions by people who felt themselves accountable to the electorate. The discovery of a human retrovirus was the acme of the viral cancer research programme's limited success. It was the sort of achievement other researchers applaud but in the cold light of a Senate Sub-Committee hearing it doesn't seem so great. Cancer research funding was in trouble. The cancer laboratories around the world had vigorously pursued every line of research which might conceivably bear fruit. These were still promising and their hands were still outstretched but the situation in the nineteen-eighties was radically different from that in the early nineteen-seventies. A massive budgetary deficit meant public spending cuts in the US and world recession meant similar actions in other countries. Cancer research had had its day. The cancer laboratories hadn't played a particularly stunning game so the politicians wanted their ball back.

AIDS arrives

Into this world of gleaming technology and dashed hopes dropped AIDS. By 1982 it became clear this was not just a local problem for homosexuals in coastal cities and the cancer laboratories began to show an interest. To return to Robert Gallo: he was head of the Laboratory of Tumor Cell Biology at the National Cancer Institute, one of twelve National Institutes of Health research establishments. Near the National Cancer Institute building in Bethesda, Maryland, is the National Institute for Allergy and Infectious Diseases into whose province the problem of AIDS would fit most appropriately. AIDS was an infectious disease, almost everyone agreed. It wasn't a cancer, anyway. If the NIH was going to look at the problem there was already an establishment designed to do just that sort of work. Moreover, at the Centers for Disease Control in Atlanta, Georgia, where the impressive epidemiological work had been done, there was a laboratory facility working on AIDS. Gallo's way into AIDS research was by no means obvious. In his own words, from an article in *Advances in Oncology*:

> I hypothesised that the infectious agent was viral in origin because Factor VIII transfusions could transmit the agent and these materials are filtered in a way that should remove bacteria and fungi and because viruses are known to be more specifically tropic for lymphocytes than are bacteria or fungi. We also proposed specifically that a retrovirus causes AIDS.
>
> In addition, the agent's apparent restricted tropism for certain target-cell types, particularly the T4 cell, was highly reminiscent of the behaviour we had observed with HTLV-I and HTLV-II. Finally, HTLV-I and HTLV-II are transmitted by blood, by sexual intercourse, and from mother to infant. In other words, the known human retroviruses were transmitted in the same way as the hypothetical agent causing AIDS.
>
> By the summer of 1982, we began to consider strongly the possibility that a T-lymphotropic retrovirus, either closely or distantly related to HTLV-I, was the cause of AIDS. We moved towards this conclusion because of several observations: M. Essex of the Harvard School of Public Health has pointed out to us that the feline leukaemia virus, a retrovirus, commonly causes immune deficiencies. The T4 tropism seen in AIDS has been observed with HTLV-I and HTLV-II. Both HTLV-I and HTLV-II can be mildly immunosuppressive. The modes of transmission of HTLV-I, HTLV-II and the putative AIDS agent were remarkably similar.

To put it another way: Robert Gallo had seen an opportunity for a new application of the techniques he had developed in his search for the leukaemia virus. If successful, this would give him another virus to add to the HTL 'family' which he had discovered.

The retrovirus hunters

In his social history of the first years of the AIDS epidemic, *And the Band Played On*, Randy Shilts stresses the importance of Don Francis at the Centers for Disease Control. This virologist worked with Max Essex on feline leukaemia and he kept Essex informed at a time when Gallo was paying scant attention to AIDS and the ball was clearly in the CDC court.

Shilts writes of Max Essex: 'He and Francis were among the small minority of scientists who believed that viruses would one day be linked to cancer and other serious human ailments. Together they had published eight articles on feline leukaemia as well as a controversial piece suggesting that some human lymphomas, leukaemias and cancers of the immune system might be linked to viral infections.'

Francis was arguing a retroviral cause for AIDS as early as June 1981. He had the ear of Essex, the premier animal retrovirologist, who had the ear of Gallo, the premier human retrovirologist. Because viruses had fallen out of fashion as putative cancer agents, there were few people in the world who had gone on to understand retroviruses. Here were three of them in professional contact.

International co-operation is the rule in medical research. Scientists who head important research facilities spend a great deal of their time flying to international conferences, reviewing papers before publication in scientific journals, playing host to foreign researchers who have visited to study new laboratory techniques. One such visit occurred in July 1982 when a researcher from the Pasteur Institute in Paris visited Gallo's lab to learn how to produce a cell culture favourable to the growth of HTLV. The theory that AIDS was caused by a variant of HTLV became known in 1982 through papers circulated via the various AIDS working parties and, of course, through simple conversation between scientists. Françoise Barré-Sinoussi, Jean-Claude Chermann and Luc Montagnier of the Virology Department at the Pasteur Institute were in an ideal position to pursue this theory. They had also been involved in the virus cancer research programme and were both intellectually and technologically equipped to detect retroviruses. Barré-Sinoussi had trained at Gallo's lab in the NCI.

One bit-part player in the drama which followed was a thirty-three-year-old Parisian homosexual fashion designer who was feeling unwell just before Christmas 1982. He called in at the La Pitié Salpêtrière hospital complaining of the now-familiar syndrome: general debility, fatigue, enlarged rubbery nodes on the neck. He had a history of several episodes of gonorrhoea and had been treated for syphilis in September 1982. He enjoyed more than fifty sexual partners a year and travelled a great deal, including travel to North America, though his last trip to New York had been in 1979.

Lab tests showed he had cytomegalovirus, Epstein-Barr virus and herpes simplex virus. The hospital had been waiting for just such a patient: almost certainly an AIDS case but one who was not so ill that his T cells were depleted and could not be encouraged to grow in culture.

A tissue sample from the lymph nodes of this patient was sent to the Pasteur Institute where Barré-Sinoussi and Chermann set about growing the lymphocytes in a culture – a complex procedure involving first anti-interferon to stop the cells from producing their own interferon and stopping the growth of a retrovirus if one were there. The next stage was to make the T cells grow, so T-cell growth factor was added, then phytohemagglutinin inducing the cells to grow larger and to divide.

About every three days there would be a test for virus – spinning the culture in a centrifuge to concentrate any virus which might be present, treating it with detergent to open up the virus and testing for reverse transcriptase. The entire procedure was, therefore, not an exploration of what unknown pathogen might be present in the lymph nodes of a man who seemed to be about to develop AIDS. The operations which were applied in the Département de Virologie of the Institut Pasteur in January 1983 were calculated to detect a retrovirus should one be present. They were not looking for the cause of AIDS, they were looking for a retrovirus.

On 25 January 1983 reverse transcriptase was found. There wasn't a great deal of reactivity to the reverse transcriptase assay and the reactivity varied widely over the next few weeks but fresh cells could be added to boost the harvest. It was definitely there.

Montagnier and his group submitted their results to the journal *Science* in April 1983 and the paper was published on 20 May – an unusually short period which indicated the urgency AIDS research had assumed in the scientific community. The paper, 'Isolation of a T-Lymphotropic Retrovirus from a Patient at Risk for Acquired Immune Deficiency Syndrome' seemed clearly to place the newly discovered virus in the Gallo family of HTLVs. Two sentences ran: 'We report here the isolation of a novel retrovirus from the lymph node of a homosexual patient with multiple lymphadenopathies. The virus appears to be a member of the human T-cell leukaemia virus (HTLV) family.'

This line was actually inserted at Gallo's suggestion when he saw an early draft of the paper as part of the 'peer review' system. The paper itself specifically contradicted the claim that there was a direct connection between the new isolate and HTLV. A comparison was made between the two proteins of the viral core of HTLV-I and the proteins of the new virus and there was no similarity. The serum of the infected patient reacted with HTLV-I infected cells which implied that the patient had come into contact with HTLV-I or something so similar to it that the patient's own antibodies could not tell the difference. When the sera of healthy donors was tested in the same way, however, the same reaction was observed. Here was certainly a novel retrovirus which in later publications (though not this one) the Montagnier group took to calling Lymphadenopathy-Associated Virus. It is worth noting their caution: 'The role of this virus in the etiology of AIDS remains to be determined,' they remarked and to note that the virus was only associated with lymphadenopathy was appropriate and commendable.

This caution contributed to the mute reception the paper received. Another significant factor was the simultaneous publication, in that same issue of *Science*, of three other papers, two from Gallo and one from Essex, associating HTLV with AIDS. The news pages of *Science* featured an article headed 'Human T-Cell Leukaemia Virus Linked to AIDS' with the sub-heading 'Patients with the new immune disease show evidence of infection by human T-cell leukaemia virus. Does the virus cause the disease?' Montagnier's work is dealt with in one sentence. As Steve Connor remarks in his thorough investigation of this for *New Scientist*: 'The very journal in which Montagnier publishes his research failed to notice the true importance of the discovery while focusing on work that turned out to be wrong.'

In keeping with the principles of scientific openness, the Pasteur Institute gave Gallo an isolate of LAV on 17 July 1983. Gallo's lab was unable to grow it. Another sample was sent on 23 September along with a contract specifying that the American lab could not use the virus to develop commercial items. The reason for this was that the French had realised the immense potential of AIDS testing kits if, as they now strongly suspected, their virus was not only associated with AIDS but was actually the cause of it. They filed for a British patent in September and a US patent in December.

Gallo wrote to a German colleague on 27 September in dismissive terms of Montagnier's work: 'I have never seen the virus that Luc Montagnier has described, and I suspect he might have a mixture of two. On the other hand, some of his data are interesting but still far from definitive. We have a total now of ten HTLV isolates from frank AIDS cases in approximately forty attempts and, again, I'm still not certain what this means.'

Despite this apparent uncertainty, Gallo was still, at least up to 12 December 1983 when a *Science* article was submitted for publication, convinced that AIDS was caused by HTLV. This article, actually published on 11 May 1984, is headed 'Antigens on HTLV-Infected Cells Recognised by Leukaemia and AIDS Sera Are Related to HTLV Viral Glycoprotein' and it attempts to demonstrate that the proteins identified on the surface of T cells infected with HTLV are 'recognised' by the antibodies in the blood of leukaemia and AIDS patients.

Before continuing with this chronology it is worth looking at exactly what was being stated when the claim was made that Human T-Cell Leukaemia Virus, or a variant of it, was causing Acquired Immune

Deficiency Syndrome. Leukaemia is characterised by an over-proliferation of leucocytes; it is a cancer – there is an uncontrolled growth. AIDS is characterised by the death of T4 cells, a particular type of leucocyte. So one disease makes them multiply and the other makes one particular type of them die. Apart from the fact that the same type of cells are involved in both diseases, what is the connection? It is impossible now to find anyone to defend the alleged connection; in 1983 while the contradiction was acknowledged it did not preclude belief in the theory. As we have seen, even Montagnier accepted an interpolation into his own paper which claimed a connection between HTLV and LAV, which that paper disproved.

It is currently difficult to find anyone to question HIV as the cause of AIDS though many express their reservations privately. It is realistic to ask how so many scientists could be wrong about HIV causing AIDS. The answer is that it doesn't take many, if a small number of specialists in the field take a particular line, specialists in other fields will accept it and generalists, and the laity, will follow suit.

Meanwhile in Cambridge, England, another former cancer resear-cher was identifying a micro-organism from the blood of an AIDS patient. Abraham Karpas of the Department of Haematological Medicine at Cambridge University Clinical School identified a virus in September 1983 and wrote a quick paper on it with an accompanying photograph of a view of these particles through an electron microscope. Karpas blames himself for not actually calling it a 'novel virus' which would have guaranteed more attention for the paper. As it was, he had some difficulty in getting the paper published, though it was accepted by *Molecular Biology in Medicine* on 14 December 1983.

This still made him, however, the second person in the world to have isolated this unusual virus from an AIDS patient and to have demonstrated the reactivity of the blood of some AIDS patients to it. Karpas later called his isolate c-LAV for 'Cambridge LAV' but did not give it this name – or any name – in the paper. Neither did he refer, even in a reference, to the work of the French team. Karpas explains that the skimpy nature of the paper was due to its having been originally submitted as a letter to *The Lancet* on 11 November 1983 only to be rejected five weeks later. He did not refer to the French because he was unable until 1984 to compare his to the French isolate and decide they were the same.

December 1983 was a busy month for all. On 14 December Mika Popovic of Gallo's laboratory received a letter from the electron microscopy laboratory they used. It dealt with the analysis of thirty-three samples of blood cells, thirty-one of them negative for viruses. The other two were both samples of LAV, in both cases the comments from the lab examining and photographing them through a microscope were the same: 'HUT 78/LAV Positive:Lentivirus. Productive lentivirus infection with all forms of virus maturation.'

HIV is probably of the lentivirus family and this is an understandable identification for the person operating the electron microscope to make. This is the proof that Gallo's lab was successfully cultivating LAV at least in December 1983. The date and the letter became vital evidence when legal action became imminent four years later. It then became known that someone in Gallo's lab had tampered with the letter quoted above to delete all reference to LAV; on the copy of the letter provided as part of the legal case, there was just a white space where in the unadulterated letter there is the reference to LAV.

Identifying the virus was one thing, growing it was quite another. Yet there had to be a sufficiently large amount of the virus cultivated for further experiments on it and, all importantly, the commercial production of kits which could test for the presence of the virus. The tendency of the virus to kill T cells in the laboratory (of which more later) meant it was very difficult to maintain a stable culture of infected cells. Eventually, Montagnier's group solved this problem by dispensing with T cells and using another kind of lymphocyte, the B cell, which had been infected with Epstein-Barr virus to make the cells multiply.

Gallo's group used a T cell line called HUT 78 in the form of a sub-group called H-9. By the end of November Gallo's group claimed to be able to cultivate sufficient quantities of the virus to be able to make clear the distinctions between it and HTLV-I. Gallo prepared for massive publication on his team's work. It is a standard rule among serious scientific publications – the breach of which can lead to 'blacklisting' by serious journals – that the results of research work should not be released prior to first publication in a scientific journal. In particular this rule is aimed at preventing a rush for publicity in the lay press with its misrepresentation and over-simplification of research results. The lay press, if it wished to report scientific findings, could do so from reports in journals with their customary caution and qualification.

In this case the usual procedure was not followed. 'Cancer Virus Tied to AIDS May Be Disclosed Soon' was the headline in the *Wall Street Journal* on 16 April 1984, 'Research Indicates AIDS Is Connected to a Cancer Virus' on 17 April in the *Washington Post*. The *New Scientist*, quoting Gallo himself, reported on 19 April:

> Researchers at America's National Cancer Institute in Bethesda, Maryland, believe they have finally tracked down the organism that causes Acquired Immune Deficiency Syndrome (AIDS). It is a virus that affects particular cells of the immune system and is called human T-cell leukaemia virus type III (HTLV-III).

There now occurred one of the strangest tableaux of the entire strange AIDS story. The Department of Health and Human Services held a press conference in Washington, DC, on 23 April to report on a new virus which had been found by Robert Gallo.

The press conference was held in a small auditorium, too small to hold the reporters and TV crews who attended. Microphones hung round the lectern like fruit weighing down a tree and scientists crowded onto the tiny stage. Secretary of Health and Human Services Margaret Heckler even introduced a scientist who wasn't there.

Gallo made a grand entrance, as described by David Black: 'He approached the podium like the only kid in the school assembly to have won a National Merit Scholarship. He was fastidiously dressed. None of Sonnabend's ratty sweaters and baggy slacks for him. He wore aviator glasses – a Hollywood touch – and his hair was rumpled, but just enough to make it look as if he had recently emerged from handling a crisis. His manner seemed to me condescending, as though he were the Keeper of Secrets obliged to deal with a world of lesser mortals.' The moral seems to be to make sure David Black is your friend before you invite him to your press conference.

Margaret Heckler acknowledged 'other discoveries . . . in different laboratories – even in different parts of the world' but the accolade was reserved for the US: 'Today we add another miracle to the long honor roll of American medicine and science.'

Heckler said the discovery of the virus would allow the development of a vaccine against AIDS which would be available by 1986. She resigned her post in 1985 and was sent to Ireland as Ambassador.

The press reported the 'discovery' straight, despite the cynicism of many reporters who knew of the French work. It is amazing that in a free society government could so manipulate the media, but there were reasons, both positive and negative, for press obeisance.

On the positive side: this was a good story for America, the sort of story readers like. AIDS had largely been an American disease so far and the story of the insidious progress of the 'gay plague' had made thrilling reading for over a year. A new angle was welcome, particularly because it was good news about American researchers in an American lab.

On the negative side: the story of a prior claim by the French team was complex, too complex for the news media to deal with in one day or, rather, the part of the day left between the end of the press conference and their deadlines. When the news editor ask 'OK, what's the story' because he or she needs to know how much space to give it, the answer 'An American scientist has found the virus which causes AIDS' is the right one. 'A press conference today announced that an American team had probably found the virus that causes AIDS but some people have been saying a French team found the virus a year ago but it didn't get much publicity,' is the wrong answer. That story cannot realistically be done in a few hours. Moreover, the electronic media relies on direct quotation from people like Heckler and Gallo and the simple, sharp quotes rule. Most Americans get their news from the electronic media and the electronic media is at the mercy of simplifiers.

An additional problem was the time difference between the US and France, should anyone wish to telephone the Pasteur Institute. There was also, perhaps, an erroneous conception that there would be a language barrier – in fact the leading characters and the press officers on the French side all speak adequate or good English.

An honourable exception to the shabby behaviour of the US media in general was the *New York Times* which, days before the press conference, featured a story in which credit for the isolation of the virus went to the Pasteur Institute. Later the *New York Times* commented on the 'fierce – and premature – fight for credit between scientists and bureaucratic sponsors of research.'

One other event occurred on 23 April: a patent was filed in the US on a test kit developed by Gallo. The prestige of coming first in the race to grow this virus was now indistinguishable from the financial gain each institute would receive if they could prove they came first. The small matter of proving that this virus actually caused the disease remained.

The fourth of May 1984 found *Science* announcing 'Strong New Candidate for AIDS Agent' on its news page with the sub-heading, 'A newly discovered member of the human T-cell leukaemia virus family is very closely linked to the immunodeficiency disease.' The leading article announced four papers in that journal, all of which appeared with Gallo's name attached and all of which dealt with an entity referred to as HTLV-III. This had been isolated from more than a third of patients with full AIDS and antibodies against it had been found in almost one hundred per cent of patients.

One of the articles contained a series of pictures taken through an electron microscope of three viruses in three stages of development: they showed virus particles budding from a cell membrane, free particles having separated from the membrane and free particles seen from a different angle. These were pictured for HTLV-I and HTLV-II showing the similarity between them. The third series of three pictures was labelled HTLV-III but it was not a picture of HTLV-III, it was a picture of the LAV isolate Montagnier had sent to Gallo. Two years later, on 18 April 1986, Gallo and others involved in the work published a correction in *Science*. Gallo explained that when he received the electron microscope pictures he simply assumed they were pictures of his HTLV. One interesting aspect of the depiction of all three together was that it showed how dissimilar LAV/HTLV-III was from the first two HTL viruses. Their cores appear pentagonal or hexagonal, the new virus looks like a rod – in fact it is cone-shaped.

The one change Gallo made to accommodate the rapidly developing understanding of the new virus was to change its name slightly from human T-cell *Leukaemia* virus to human T-cell *Lymphotropic* virus indicating a tropism (affinity for) T cells.

The proof that LAV/HTLV-III was not of the HTLV family came when the viruses underwent nucleic acid sequencing through the end of 1984. This is a procedure for working out the genetic structure of a virus. It was therefore possible to be definitive: the new virus does not have sufficient similarity to the HTLVs for them to belong to the same family.

This had long been believed to be the case and was hardly a surprise. The level of similarity between HTLV-III and LAV did surprise even case-hardened scientists, however.

Reverse transcriptase does not do a perfect job; when it converts RNA to DNA there are mutations occurring which change the virus so each isolate should be quite different. To put it another way: there should be sufficient similarities to demonstrate they are the same virus but unless they are clones, meaning they came from the same culture, there should also be differences. The differences between LAV and HTLV-III were insignificant. The differences between them were no greater than between clones of the same isolate grown in the same culture.

Gallo said this might have occurred because both isolates were, by chance, from mutual sexual partners. This would mean Montagnier's patient with lymphadenopathy would have had to have had sex with someone in New York in 1979 and three or four years later that person in New York would have had to have a sample of serum taken in which there was unchanged virus.

Another test for the genetic similarity of viruses came up with the same answer: of twelve different viruses studied by restriction mapping (measuring specific elements of the DNA rather than all the genes), all were different except LAV and HTLV-III.

The evidence, then, that LAV and HTLV-III were the same and that Montagnier got there first is in four parts: First, it is not questioned that Gallo's lab received isolates of Montagnier's virus twice while they did not reciprocate. Secondly, there seems to have been some tampering with letters to delete a reference to the fact that LAV was growing in Gallo's cell line.

The pictures in *Science* with Gallo's four HTLV-III papers are also telling. Gallo claims he had pictures of his isolate as early as February 1983 giving him obvious precedence over the French. But this comment, as Steve Connor notes in *New Scientist*, 'does not explain why, if he could photograph the HTLV-III virus in February 1983, he waited until May 1984 to publish pictures of the virus and even then made the mistake of publishing pictures not of HTLV-III but of Montagnier's LAV.'

Finally, the two most sensitive methods of analysis of viral genetic material show the two isolates to be remarkably similar.

This acrimonious dispute between different teams of researchers was increasingly personified in public by the personalities of the men involved – Montagnier Gallic and aloof; Gallo hurt, defensive, emotional. Just as they had been obliged to race to be first to isolate and cultivate this new virus, now they had to defend steadfastly the importance of their discovery. They had no time for quiet reflection and could hardly have turned round to their governments, their journalists, their lawyers, to say: 'Sorry, we got it wrong, back to the drawing board.'

The lawyers were playing an increasingly significant part. Despite Montagnier's group having filed for US patents on the test for antibodies to the new virus before Gallo's group did, the US Patent and Trademark Office awarded Gallo a patent on 28 May 1985. The Pasteur Institute heard nothing and had to file a complaint before the US claims court. This action, one of three which made the picture of LAV/HTLV-III yet more murky, claimed Gallo had infringed the written agreement not to use the samples of LAV for commercial purposes.

The second was the action over the patent rights to the test kit. The US Patent and Trademark Office accepted Montagnier's prior claim in May 1986 and made the French the 'senior party', which meant they had prior claim and Gallo's team had to prove they were first. The third action concerned the US Freedom of Information Act and the non-disclosure of documents from Gallo's laboratory which the French lawyers needed to see.

The legal dispute between these institutes does not affect the central question of this book, namely whether or not the virus they isolated is actually the cause of AIDS. For this reason there will not be an account of the progress of the dispute. Most importantly, the cases demonstrated how much was riding on this virus in terms of national kudos, personal prestige for the researchers and, not least, cash. The market for AIDS testing kits based on this virus was worth $100 million a year.

The dispute was settled in April 1987 in terms which meant there were two patents on the test kits. Eighty per cent of the royalties collected by both sides on their test kits were to go to a new foundation based in the

US researching into AIDS. The foundation, with three French-appointed and three American-appointed trustees, was to award grants to scientists working on human retroviruses – keeping it in the family, so to speak.

Part of the agreement the two parties signed was a statement that they agreed to be bound by a particular historical interpretation of the events leading to the isolation of the virus. An official history was written and all parties had to 'agree to be bound by such scientific history and further agree that they shall not make or publish any statements which would or could be construed as contradicting or compromising the integrity of the said history.' If scientific fraud is the worst professional crime a scientist can conceive of, probably the worst for a historian is the rewriting of history to accommodate some establishment view.

The name of the virus

The International Committee on the Taxonomy of Viruses declared in May 1986 that the virus should not be called by its previous names, it was becoming confusing and was tying up scientific nomenclature in titles related to national prestige. It was named HIV by the subcommittee working on it. The letters stood for Human Immunodeficiency Virus, thus following the usual nomenclature of microbes which is to state first which species it infects, then what it is said to do, then what kind of a microbe it is. All on the subcommittee accepted this except Robert Gallo and Max Essex but, to everyone else in the scientific world, HIV it became.

Another reason for the unification of the names was the number of people who had by now isolated it and given it their own title. Another cancer researcher, Jay Levy in California, had isolated what he called ARV – AIDS-associated retrovirus. The Centers for Disease Control had tried to please all of the people all of the time by calling theirs LAV/HTLV-III-CDC-151 but mercifully it failed to thrive in culture. A German team also had an AIDS-associated virus. If HIV is not the cause of AIDS, how did so many well-qualified scientists come up with the same microbe? Surely this is an indication that the original isolation of a microbe in a patient by Montagnier's group was correct – everyone else confirmed it, after all.

The fact that more than one laboratory can find the virus is indeed proof that it is there, but that has never been questioned by the critics who say HIV does not cause AIDS. Not only is it there in many AIDS patients, they say, but it is also there in many healthy people who do not have and are not going to have AIDS. It was found, the claim runs, because it was looked for.

This is why Robert Gallo assumes such central importance despite the probability that he did not isolate HIV first and that even his early isolates were 'contaminated' with the virus sent from France. Gallo's work, at a time when other scientists had virtually abandoned the field, led directly to human retroviruses. He and his lab developed the techniques possible for detecting them, he put human retroviruses on the microbiological map. When he suggested in 1982 that AIDS might be caused by another human retrovirus he had already earned some prestige as the discoverer of HTLV-I. Other laboratories followed the lead he gave both in the quest for a retrovirus and the techniques used to detect and culture one.

John Wyke of the Beatson Institute in Glasgow, Scotland, has as much experience as anyone in hunting viruses – again from the virus/cancer research programme. He said:

> The favoured approach is to look for something which is like something you know already. You say, this disease is similar in some ways to another disease and we know the cause of that so let's look for something of the same family. Of course you use the same techniques.
>
> If you don't know what is there at all, it is very difficult in virology to look for something. What techniques do you use?
>
> Of course there have been mistakes in the past, viruses have been identified as the cause of a disease incorrectly, but everyone is aware of the possibility of these mistakes and is on guard against them.

To repeat Gallo's remark: 'We had the technology to perform sensitive assays for retroviruses and for culturing T lymphocytes *in vitro*, so using it seemed to be the logical first step in our search for the AIDS agent.'

A standard principle of science is replication – this means that work in one laboratory should be able to be duplicated by another.

Once one laboratory has achieved something, like the isolation of a new microbe, it is incumbent upon other labs to validate or invalidate the work. To do this they have to use the same instruments and the same techniques, to measure their quantities of sera and reagents in the same amounts, to spin substances in a centrifuge for the same amount of time at the same speed. It is this need for replication, incidentally, which makes scientific journals so difficult for lay people to read. The basic concepts are intellectually accessible to anyone of above-average intelligence; it is the technical terminology necessary so other labs can replicate the work which is impenetrable without years of study.

The other labs proved, using Gallo's own techniques, that there were retroviruses in the tissues of at least some AIDS patients. Perhaps it was faulty technique which meant they failed to find them in the tissues of all AIDS patients. So the original work was confirmed, and the dispute started as to which family the new virus belonged to and who had found it first. No one seemed to heed the warning in an editorial in the *New Scientist*: 'The scientific journals should beware of being steamrollered by scientists who are rushing forward so quickly that they do not have the time needed to make the usual series of painstaking experiments to confirm their original thought.'

The virus hunters

If a virus were sought for the cause of a disease and misidentified as the cause for the first time in the case of AIDS, this would be remarkable. In fact this error is far from being without precedent. Viruses are 'flavour of the century' just as bacteria were a hundred years ago. Since the nineteen-forties we have had electron microscopes which can be used to see viruses just as in the nineteenth century there were optical microscopes which could be used to see bacteria. Concepts adjust to fit the technology available to them. At the end of the nineteenth century every disease was caused by a bacteria. Today every disease is caused by a virus.

A few examples: five years were spent hunting a virus for the cause of Lyme disease, an inflammatory condition like arthritis. Originally described in Lyme, Connecticut, where many residents are affected, the disease causes swelling in knees and other large joints with chills, fever and headache associated with the condition. It is passed from animals such as deer via their ticks to humans. The textbook in which I have just looked up the condition (dated 1983) notes it is 'believed to be transmitted by an unidentified tickborne virus.' It was eventually identified by Willy Burgdorfer as being caused by a corkscrew-shaped bacteria called a spirochete which was named Borrelia burgdorferi in his honour.

Similarly, a distinctive form of pneumonia was identified by clinicians but its cause was a subject of speculation which always hinged on a viral cause until an organism called Mycoplasma pneumoniae was isolated. Mycoplasma is a curious genus of micro-organisms. They are able to be grown in an artificial medium in the absence of a cell line and are therefore not viruses, for viruses cannot replicate outside a cell. They are distinguished from bacteria, however, in that they do not have a rigid cell wall.

In some cases, the very means used to attempt to detect a virus has destroyed the actual agent in culture, thus making it close to impossible to detect the agent. The case of Legionnaires' disease aptly demonstrates this. The 1976 convention of the American Legion was held in the Bellevue-Stratton Hotel, Philadelphia. Within a few days scores of the delegates became ill with chills, fevers, dry coughs and muscle pains. There were 182 cases of this odd pneumonia, with 29 deaths.

The air-conditioning system was immediately suspected as most of the cases were associated with congregating in the hotel lobby. Moreover, other cases occurred in pedestrians in the street outside who had not been associated with the hotel, the so-called Broad Street disease. The only thing the street had in common with the hotel was that the same air had been in both places, moved around by the air-conditioning system.

Researchers set out to find their virus. No virus could be found in lung tissue taken from the victims. Diseased tissue was injected into guinea pigs with unhelpful results: some died, some stayed healthy and the virus couldn't be found in the lung tissue of either group.

Another attempt at growing the virus involved injecting infected tissue into hens' eggs after antibiotics had been used to kill any bacteria which might grow in the eggs and contaminate the experiment. But they still couldn't grow that virus.

Finally Joe McDade, a thirty-six-year-old research microbiologist at the Centers for Disease Control, went back to the slides of diseased tissue which had previously failed to yield up the secret of the microbe. This time he found it, but it wasn't a virus, it was a bacterium which was named Legionella pneumophilia. Once one bacterium had been identified, more followed and now there are ten sub-groups of Legionella pneumophilia and eighteen other similar organisms including Legionella micdadei, named in honour of Joe McDade.

Legionella lives in air-conditioning systems, cooling towers, showers – wherever there is dirty water which can then find itself sprayed and inhaled by susceptible people. The chain of events necessary to cause illness is interesting and, in its complex interplay of social, micro-biological and medical factors, sheds some light on AIDS. The water needs to be still at some times and not frequently changed: there has to be a reservoir, however small, of dirty water. The bacteria must come into contact with it. It has to be turned into a spray. It has to be inhaled by people. There have been cases in young people but most are in middle-aged to elderly men with a most commonly occurring age of fifty-seven. Death rate is highest in those who already have a heart or lung condition, are immunosuppressed or have diabetes. Smoking is also a risk factor.

We thus have a peculiarly modern disease. It is relatively recently in human history that air-conditioners and showers have existed. It is also relatively recent that people who have the variety of problems which predispose to infection by Legionella should stay alive and active.

Once the agent was understood, as in AIDS, retrospective diagnoses began to be made. It is now realised that 'Pontiac fever', in 1967 when ninety-five per cent of the staff at a US Health Department suffered breathing difficulties, was caused by Legionella. There was a leak between the ducts of the evaporating cooler system and the ventilation system in which the bacteria were growing.

Besides this complexity, there were other problems in the way of the most dedicated researcher: there was no good animal model. Laboratory animals are notoriously bad models for human disease. How could a guinea pig duplicate the physical condition of a fifty-seven-year-old American man who has mild diabetes and smokes? In what quantities should the microbes be given to the lab animal? Which animal should be used? Mycobacterium leprae, which causes leprosy, will not infect any known animal but man and the armadillo.

A cell culture can be used instead of an animal but how should the cell culture be prepared? In the early CDC search, antibiotics were used to clear the way for the culture of the all-important virus. Of course, the bacteria which were the cause of the epidemic were destroyed immediately.

Finally, there is the problem of size. It is possible to look so closely for viruses at magnifications of 100,000 times that larger particles are simply missed: a classic case of not seeing the wood for the trees.

The virus hunt of all virus hunts has been that quest for the virologist's grail, the virus which causes human cancer. In this, of course, the most common cancers are the cancers it would be most desirable to link to a virus. The equation runs 'cancer plus virus equals vaccine plus Nobel Prize'. The lack of success has been overwhelming.

The case of breast cancer is an interesting one, particularly because it received media attention in the nineteen-seventies through the premature announcement of promising lab results.

Viruses do seem to play a role in the mammary tumours of mice. The virus is passed on in milk to the mouse's young. When virus-like particles were found in human breast milk, scientists warned women with a family history of breast cancer not to breast-feed their children because of the possibility of passing on the cancer virus from mother to daughter.

For a series of commonsense reasons, this was bad advice. One is epidemiological: breast cancer rates are low in countries where breast-feeding is common but are increasing in countries like the US where breast-feeding rates are low. Another is genetic: breast cancer occurs equally in women with a family history of breast cancer on both the male and the female side of the family. Another reason is biochemical: human milk may inactivate viruses. If so, it might inactivate a putative cancer virus. The last point is statistical: the 'cancer viruses' occur with almost as much frequency in healthy women as in those with breast cancer.

Stated in this way, the arguments against a simple connection between viruses and breast cancer seem overwhelming, but many labs, many mice, many scientists and much money were channelled into this question in the seventies. In his review of the evidence Nurul Sarkar of Memorial Sloan-Kettering Cancer Center, New York, says:

> The evidence for a viral involvement in human breast cancer is contradictory and inconclusive (and) scientists have a special responsibility not to raise public hopes for a cure or a prophylaxis for breast cancer based on suggestive rather than conclusive data. In the past many scientists have expressed their own beliefs as if they were proven fact. . . . I think that it is important to remember that there are fundamental differences between humans and laboratory strains of animals. We should be able to accept the fact that human breast cancer may not be caused by a virus. An open-minded attitude on this question will provide the mental freedom that is essential to creative and innovative research into the cause of human breast cancer.

Inevitably, once the human retroviruses were described, researchers started looking for them in breasts and found them. Scientists at the University of Liverpool, England, reported in January 1988 a study of tissue from thirty-two women with breast cancer and twenty-seven healthy controls. Reverse transcriptase activity was found in thirty-one of the patients and three of the control group.

Examination through an electron microscope found evidence of the virus in cells of the walls of blood vessels but not in cells of the developing tumour. The researchers admitted that some of the 'viruses' may have been misidentified natural particles ('coated vesicles').

Interestingly from the point of view of anyone questioning the HIV hypothesis, the scientists reporting in *The Lancet* suggest a mechanism by which a retrovirus could be located in a person already immune-suppressed: 'It is possible that the virus is present in the monocyte series of cells only, plays no part in the development of the malignancy, and has merely been unmasked by the accidental immunosuppressive effect of the tumour.'

Other diseases in which retroviruses have recently been sought and found are non-A non-B hepatitis and Kawasaki disease, in which children suffer fevers, rashes and swelling of the lymph nodes.

A virus a year

If HIV is a passenger along with many other passenger viruses, it should be possible to find not only HIV but also other retroviruses. It is indeed true that now the technology is in place to detect retroviruses, laboratories all over the world are coming up with new ones. It was, in fact, the presence of more than one retrovirus in the bodies of patients which contributed to the confusion about whether 'the' virus in AIDS patients was really HTLV-I. Even in Montagnier's first presentation in September 1982 he noted that fourteen per cent of his AIDS patients had been infected with HTLV-I as well as the new virus.

In 1986 Montagnier's group isolated another retrovirus, now referred to as HIV-2, from a patient in West Africa. As *Newsweek* put it: 'At first the French doctors were doubly mystified. The thirty-two-year-old man was clearly suffering from AIDS. Yet he had come to Paris from the Cape Verde islands off the coast of Senegal, thousands of miles from Central Africa, from where the vast majority of the continent's AIDS victims come. Even more curious was the fact that routine blood tests showed he had produced no antibodies to HIV, the human immunodeficiency virus that causes AIDS.'

One avenue of approach would have been: 'therefore re-examine the HIV hypothesis' but researchers instead went on to isolate another form of HIV. People with both HIV-2 and AIDS have been hard to come by – more than half of a group of thirty-nine prostitutes in Guinea-Bissau have HIV-2 but none have AIDS, for example.

HIV-1 and HIV-2 are about forty per cent identical though many people who believe that HIV-1 causes AIDS, like Max Essex, have doubts about HIV-2. Essex said: 'From my perspective it doesn't have epidemic potential, if it did we would have seen it by now.'

Max Essex was involved in another AIDS virus discovery, one which went badly wrong. In pursuit of the elusive connection between the African green monkey and AIDS, Essex in his laboratory at Harvard examined isolates of viruses from both African green monkey and West African humans. Eureka! They were the same! The family tree of how the virus jumped the 'species barrier' could finally be drawn, the proof of the connection between the monkeys and the human disease, long prophesied, was finally at hand. The new isolate was proudly labelled HTLV-IV (Essex had never accepted the change of 'AIDS virus' nomenclature to HIV).

There had been questions, and sneers, about laboratory contamination but the clinching argument came when 'genetic mapping' of the isolate took place. The 'HTLV-IV' turned out to be ninety-nine per cent genetically identical not only with an African green monkey isolate but also with a macaque virus in the same laboratory at the Harvard School of Public Health where the work was done.

Scientists from the New England Regional Primate Center at Harvard Medical School clarified the question when they explained in *Nature* that they isolated what they called SIV (simian immunodeficiency virus) from macaques in September 1984. Subsequently they gave Max Essex a sample of the isolate in a HUT-78 cell line. It was worked on in the same lab as that in which work with African green monkey and HIV were continuing. There was only one retrovirus and it was from the macaques; it then contaminated the other cultures in some unexplained way.

Other human retroviruses coming to the fore included SBL 6669 V-2 from the Swedish Karolinska Institute (1986) and HTLV-V from the Universities of Rome and L'Aquila (1987).

Controversy was caused in June 1987 when Gallo announced another human retrovirus at the world conference on AIDS in Washington, DC. A 'distant relative' of HIV-1 and HIV-2 had been found in Nigerian patients with AIDS-like symptoms.

February 1988 saw Max Essex announcing he had found populations in the Ivory Coast and in Senegal where in a total of eighty-one AIDS patients, twenty-nine did not have antibodies to HIV-1 or HIV-2. The report noted that he 'does not rule out the possibility that there is a third human retrovirus causing AIDS in West Africa'.

The Fourth International Conference on AIDS in Stockholm in June 1988 was presented with reports of HIV-3. A new virus was isolated from a pregnant woman in Cameroon. She was healthy but her husband 'showed early signs of AIDS'. One of the Belgian discoverers said the new virus was forty per cent similar to HIV-1.

It seems likely retroviruses will continue to be discovered at a steady rate in the foreseeable future.

Research contracts

Not everyone accepted the hypothesis that HIV causes AIDS but the dissenting voices were drowned in the clamour of competing claims for precedence and applications for research grants to study the new microbiological marvel.

Alan Cantwell was one who immediately realised that the HIV hypothesis did not answer the questions AIDS posed. He said: 'Scientists clearly avoided the issue of what was causing Kaposi's sarcoma in the [HIV antibody] negative patients. I wondered how a new virus could possibly cause a century-old form of cancer. There was absolutely no direct link between [HIV] infection and the development of Kaposi's sarcoma. This fact didn't seem to deter most AIDS experts who insisted that the new virus was the sole cause of AIDS.'

Cantwell runs through some of the theories which persisted about the cause of AIDS, then notes dolefully: 'I continued to get some of my research work on bacteria in AIDS published in medical journals, although it was increasingly clear to me that medical editors were becoming more and more unresponsive to any research which did not conform to the idea of the new virus as the sole cause of AIDS.'

Cantwell was spotting interesting bacteria in the skin tumours of Kaposi's sarcoma and in lung tissue affected with Pneumocystis pneumonia. Of course, he might have been mistaken in what he saw or the bacteria might be harmless, but one would at least have thought it merited consideration.

Most research which did not comply with the HIV hypothesis was simply ignored. Joe Sonnabend suffered a worse fate.

In 1983 he set up a journal titled *AIDS Research* which was a forum 'for basic research and clinical observations on Acquired Immuno-deficiency Syndrome'. It used direct reproduction methods so that articles could be distributed fast.

AIDS Research did not ignore the HIV hypothesis. Some of its articles were directly within the field of the hypothesis, some questioned it or sections of it. Others simply dealt with new methods of treatment. There were articles about the association between AIDS and syphilis and treatment of disseminated cytomegalovirus infection and the effect of rectal insemination on laboratory rabbits.

There were twenty-one people on the board of *AIDS Research* when it was still an independent journal in the autumn of 1986. The Burroughs Wellcome Company then began to fund the journal, presumably out of the profits it was making from AZT, the AIDS drug, which will be discussed in more detail later in this book. The journal was renamed *AIDS Research and Human Retroviruses*. There were nine articles in the first edition in 1987, seven of them about HIV and two about other retroviruses alleged to be linked to it. There were fifty people on the new editorial board, only two of them had been on the *AIDS Research* board. Joe Sonnabend, of course, had gone.

Robert Gallo became a household name as few other scientists have done. He enjoyed public acclaim from people who could not know enough to criticise him and surrounded himself at the National Institutes of Health with colleagues whose respect bordered on adoration. One press officer told me Gallo was 'the complete Renaissance man' and Sam Broder, another cancer researcher, said: 'Gallo is one of the paradigmatic figures of the twentieth century. He's influenced things in our daily lives to an incalculable degree. Einstein, Freud – I'd put him on a list like that, I really would.'

A more balanced picture of Gallo was featured in the magazine *Advances in Oncology*, noting he has served for fifteen years as Chief of the Laboratory of Tumor Cell Biology, Departmental Therapeutics Program, National Cancer Institute. 'In that position he has transformed what might otherwise have been a relatively unnoticed basic research facility into an ignescent force in the battle against AIDS.'

Or maybe not. 'Without Robert Gallo there would have been no HIV' is a great compliment if he is right. If he is wrong, it is a great curse.

Coda

As always, what did not happen is as significant as what did. Remember the fashion designer, the thirty-three-year-old Parisian homosexual who was feeling unwell just before Christmas 1982? Doctor Willy Rosenbaum took a sample of tissue from his enlarged lymph nodes and sent it to Montagnier's groups at the Pasteur Institute. What happened to that patient? This was the most famous AIDS patient in history, the one from whom the 'AIDS virus' was isolated, which gave the discovery to Montagnier. It was the virus which was sent to Gallo's laboratory and which was almost identical to the one Gallo claimed he had found. Five years later that patient was still alive and well and living in Paris.

When Willy Rosenbaum talked to me in July 1988, five and a half years after the patient had been to see him with lymphadenopathy, he assured me that the patient was very well. So, he added as a matter of interest, was the other patient whose tissue was taken at the same time to demonstrate that he had antibodies to the virus.

It is possible to over-interpret this information. As Willy Rosenbaum said: 'The majority of patients who are infected have no AIDS.' Even according to the establishment view, it is possible to accept the presence of the virus without the clinical disease. I feel it is more of symbolic importance: within five years the most famous HIV patient in the world did not develop AIDS.

Four

HIV Challenged

THERE IS A STORY that Peter Duesberg once found himself in the witness box in a court. Asked to describe his profession he said he was a virologist. The court didn't feel fully enlightened at this and asked, by way of clarification, who the world leader in this field was. 'I am,' said Duesberg. The judge noted that this might be so, but it wasn't terribly modest to say so. 'But I am under oath,' said Duesberg.

Peter Duesberg must have been one of those infuriating kids who was good at everything when he was at school. People like him with a command of literature and languages as well as his own science subjects invariably anger mediocrities. More than once I have been told Duesberg is 'too clever by half'.

Born in Germany in 1936, he took his PhD in chemistry at Frankfurt University in 1963 and almost immediately was snatched up by the University of California at Berkeley, where he has been since 1964, as Professor of the Department of Molecular Biology since 1973. His background in chemistry is one of the things the AIDS researchers, who all have medical degrees, hold against him. How could a biochemist have the temerity to challenge a medical doctor? Doctors, as every patient knows, do not like to be contradicted, regardless of the facts.

Duesberg once remarked: 'Why are MDs so resistant to challenge to their authority? Why won't doctors like any other scientists accept the possibility they may be wrong? In any other discipline you put a theory, then you see it challenged and you discuss it, but not with MDs. If you challenge their theory, they take it as a personal insult.'

It should be sufficient, without citing Duesberg's several hundred scientific papers, to note that he has been working as a virologist since 1963 and in 1986 he was elected to the prestigious National Academy of Sciences. If anyone knows his way around viruses it is Peter Duesberg.

As Robert Gallo said of him when introducing him to a scientific audience in 1984: 'He began working with retroviruses around 1966 and he was among the first, perhaps even the very first, to characterise their structural proteins. He was involved in the first work that provided a genetic map of retroviruses. Surely, this is one of the most important of his many biochemical contributions, that is, the order of the genes *gag, pol* and *env*, and some aspects of the nature of their nucleotide sequences. We now know that this fundamental result is applicable to all retroviruses, including HTLV-I, II and III (HIV).'

Gallo further remarked on Duesberg's personality, that he 'is a man of extraordinary energy, unusual honesty, enormous sense of humour, and a rare critical sense. This critical sense often makes us look twice, then a third time, at a conclusion many of us believed to be foregone.'

Clearly Duesberg had been controversial before, to the chagrin of some of his colleagues and obviously to the delight of others. John Wyke said: 'Peter is a polemicist, he will pitch a line and stick to it through thick and thin.' In 1985 he challenged one aspect of the theory of 'onc' or cancer-causing genes on which a great deal of his own reputation was based.

His interest in HIV came when he did what the head of every other well-equipped cancer laboratory did in the early nineteen-eighties – he looked at the literature on HIV to determine whether he could put together a research proposal to investigate some aspect of this virus and attract some of that pot of gold over to Berkeley. He became increasingly disconcerted with the published papers: none of them gave adequate evidence of the biochemical activity of HIV in patients or of any link between the virus and AIDS except the existence of the virus in a latent form in many AIDS patients. 'I could not write a fundable project in AIDS research assuming that this virus is the cause of AIDS and that I were a reviewer of the grant application,' he said.

He chatted about this with scientific colleagues, never receiving the information which would adequately prove there was more than mere association between HIV and the disease. Finally the editor of one of the world's major cancer journals, *Cancer Research*, asked him to write a paper on his views about HIV and retroviruses in general.

It took nine months to write and Duesberg considers he must have read every major paper on HIV and not a few of the minor ones. He references 278 papers. The article, 'Retroviruses as Carcinogens and Pathogens: Expectation and Reality' runs to twenty-one pages – a prodigious length for an academic paper. Published in the March 1987 edition of *Cancer Research*, two-thirds of its argument covers animal and human retroviruses in general – including HTLV-I – and the question of whether they are capable of causing illness. How similar are they to the animal retroviruses which do cause cancer? What structure and what mechanism do they have which will allow them to cause cancer?

In the last third of the paper, he turns his attention to HIV and skilfully dismantles the flawed reasoning behind its allegedly causal relationship with AIDS.

Low levels of HIV in patients

If HIV were a powerful pathogen, it could reasonably be expected that high levels of virus would be found in people with AIDS. Given the attention HIV has received, it might be expected that laboratories would be testing the levels of virus in the blood of AIDS patients and healthy carriers night and day. Actually, Duesberg could find no record in the considerable scientific literature of any measurement of what is referred to as the 'virus titre'. This is a measurement of the parts of virus per millilitre (thousandths of a litre) of blood.

'There are probably tens of thousands of papers in the literature of this virus and not one has reported the titre,' he said.

Duesberg asked Jay Levy about the titres and was told they were between 0 and 10^2 per millilitre. Not to become too technical, it would probably be simplest to see this level of virus in relation to another viral disease. Hepatitis viruses reach titres of 10^{12-13} before they cause hepatitis. The body has to be awash with them. Up to that point they do not cause disease.

How, asks Duesberg, does a virus which infects as few as one in 100,000 cells cause a generalised infection?

The Chiron corporation in Emeryville, just outside San Francisco, produces a range of biological products including HIV testing kits. They are currently part of the great competition to find a vaccine against HIV. Their economic viability, therefore, depends in a large part on detailed knowledge of HIV. Their Director of Virology, Dino Dina, was bracingly honest about the limitations of their knowledge. He said:

In general, people have not been able to detect any substantial levels of virus in AIDS patients and that has been one of the most puzzling aspects of the viral infection.

Between one in ten thousand and one in a hundred thousand cells in the peripheral blood of patients can be shown to be infected at any given time.

More recent results have shown that alternative cells to the T cells have been identified as a target for the virus, these are the macrophages which are also part of the immune system and they can be a large reservoir for the virus, particularly in the initial phases of the infection. But even then the number of cells is very small and the amount of circulating viruses is essentially so low that it cannot be practically detected by most tests available today.

Duesberg takes the argument a stage further by asking what the situation would be if the virus were virulent and did kill cells. It is present in so few cells, he says, that even if it were to kill its share of T cells every twenty-four to forty-eight hours, 'it would hardly ever match or beat the natural rate of T-cell regeneration.'

There is a vast amount of 'redundancy' in the body: over-production of cells so it is possible to continue to function even after many cells have been put out of action. Therefore, though alcohol excess destroys brain cells, Duesberg laughed, 'we can go to an orgy one night, a few thousand brain cells go, another night and the same thing. You have to go to an orgy every night for a long time for this to have any noticeable effect.'

We wouldn't be around representing essentially a three billion-year tradition of life if we could die from losing one per cent or 0.01 per cent of our T cells, even every forty-eight hours.

We can detect viruses at that level because biotechnology has advanced so much, but we can't prove that they could be pathogenic under such conditions because no virus, no microbe ever is.

The idea of a virus killing so few cells and killing the whole body this way is like trying to conquer China by shooting five Chinese soldiers every day – you would have to go a long way before you'd won.

Logically, we would expect there to be more virus in the blood of patients seriously ill with AIDS as compared with those who are only HIV carriers. To quote from Duesberg's *Cancer Research* paper: 'There is no evidence that the virus titre or the level of virus infiltration increases during the acute phase of the disease. It is probably for this reason that cells from AIDS patients must be propagated several weeks in culture, apart from the host's immune system before either spontaneous or chemically induced virus expression may occur.'

Duesberg also notes that the virus is absent from Kaposi's sarcoma, and there are similarly low levels in the brains of people with AIDS-associated brain disease and in the lungs of people suffering from Pneumocystis carinii pneumonia.

Dino Dina tended to confirm Duesberg's position, even though he holds the view that HIV does cause AIDS. Asked if the virus level rises as the disease becomes acute, he said: 'No, in fact as the disease progresses the number of cells that can harbour the virus diminishes because of the immune suppression and it becomes increasingly difficult to demonstrate the presence of the virus in those patients.'

What happens to this virus? Does it disappear simultaneously from T cells, Langerhans' cells, macrophages and lung cells? Is there a precedent in any other infection for this vanishing act? Or is it just that it was only there in tiny quantities in the first place?

It is accepted that T helper cells decline as AIDS progresses and that HIV can be found in T helper cells. But the death of T helper cells seems to be reducing the amount of virus, i.e. the body's decline from AIDS, far from releasing massive quantities of virus to further ravage the system, seems to be killing off the HIV as well. It certainly seems from this evidence to be a passenger virus rather than one which is relentlessly slaying cells then going on to cause fatal disease.

How do scientists find themselves in the position of chasing viruses which are in such tiny quantities in patients? Normally they don't bother. Abraham Karpas said:

It depends on the technology of the laboratory how many AIDS patients we can recover the virus from. Potentially one should be able to recover it practically from every person who is infected.

In fact this doesn't always happen because it depends on the sensitivity of the test used in a particular laboratory and also it's a very time consuming business. There is no real time to spend several weeks to a month to look for a virus while if you do tests for antibodies you can tell within two hours whether a person is infected or not.

Duesberg would argue that this difficulty of isolating the virus confirms the extremely low virus titres in AIDS patients. Moreover, the isolation figures he uses come from tests performed at the laboratories of the National Institutes of Health in Maryland by people who support the HIV hypothesis.

When looking for the genetic material of HIV, a technique called molecular hybridisation is used. One HIV gene can be detected in ten or one hundred and a cell contains a million genes. To put it another way: the quest for the genetic material of HIV must be sensitive enough to detect less than one gene in a million to ten million genes. With these tests, the genetic material of the virus (proviral DNA, to be specific) has been found in only fifteen per cent of patients. If it is not detected in the other eighty-five per cent, that means there is less of it or it is not there. The latent virus – not replicating, just existing – can be found in fifty per cent of AIDS patients.

Newer and more sophisticated methods of investigation only made the problem of looking for HIV worse. Helga Rübsamen-Waigmann subjected T cells from ninety-one AIDS patients to the most extreme battery of tests. Her lab work was beyond criticism, yet three of these patients consistently refused to yield up virus.

The most advanced technique available, called PCR (polymerase chain reaction), is able to find one DNA molecule in a million, then multiply the target molecule more than a billion times in order that it can be studied. Even with this technique, four out of eleven people with antibodies to HIV but no identifiable virus still gave a negative test.

This sort of problem has long been a matter of discussion among the AIDS establishment and their opponents alike. The opponents are not reverent about it. *New York Native* printed the 'AIDS Jokes':

Q: What's the only virus that is there if you can't find it?
A: HIV.
Q: What's the difference between HIV and God?
A: You can always find God in an AIDS patient.

The HIV antibody test

With such low levels of the virus in AIDS patients, how can AIDS be diagnosed by people who believe the theory that HIV causes the disease? In the absence of a test for the virus, they must test for evidence that the virus has been there. The test which is widely known as 'the AIDS test' is a test for antibodies to the virus: proof that a person had been in contact with the virus and that their immune system had produced antibodies to protect itself.

Duesberg said:

The best evidence that the virus is associated with AIDS patients is antibody to the virus which is at best an indirect test. In fact, it's almost an argument against the virus causing the disease because typically antibody to a virus means vaccination, protection.

It is effective too, it is so effective that the virus titre is undetectable. It takes a very expensive laboratory to activate the virus and grow it in a cell culture.

The argument of those who support the HIV theory of the cause of AIDS is that the virus is so powerful, the antibodies cannot kill it.

Abraham Karpas goes one step further and argues for the existence of neutralising and non-neutralising antibodies: those which will contain the virus and those which will not. The people who do not develop AIDS have neutralising antibodies which work against the virus, the people who do develop the syndrome have non-neutralising antibodies. The results of his work should make an interesting contribution to the AIDS debate.

It is paradoxical that the presence of HIV is detected by looking for antibodies to HIV because the only reason the test can work is that the antibodies from a patient are attacking the HIV. To explain the test rather crudely: blood from the person being tested is put in a test tube with some of the virus itself (which has been grown in a cell culture). If the person has been in contact with HIV before, this new contact will make the blood produce antibodies which will adhere to the HIV. But they will look exactly the same. In order to render the reaction visible, therefore, a substance which will adhere only to HIV antibodies has to be dropped into the test tube. But it must not only stick to the antibodies, it must go through a chemical change which will make it change colour when it sticks to the antibodies. The degree to which it has changed colour is the degree to which antibodies to HIV exist in the blood. This is measured by a laser connected to a computer which will give a numerical value to each degree of colour change.

It is even more paradoxical that people with a low level of antibodies to HIV are considered to be at low risk from AIDS. Duesberg wrote in the *Cancer Research* paper, that the HIV theory 'fails to explain why active antiviral immunity, which includes neutralising antibody and which effectively prevents virus spread and expression, would not prevent the virus from causing a fatal disease.' He then comments rather coyly: 'It is also unexpected that AIDS patients are capable of mounting an apparently highly effective antiviral immunity, although immunodeficiency is the hallmark of the disease.'

Duesberg is criticised for his claim that the existence of antibodies shows the patient is putting up a good defence against attack from HIV. His opponents cite examples of diseases where antibodies are present but the disease enjoys a resurgence after a period of latency. Herpes is a frequent example. Patients with herpes have antibodies to their herpes virus. The virus is, most of the time, not causing an outbreak of herpes sores, it is remaining latent in the nerve fibres. But the antibodies cannot be sufficient to hold it in check because it periodically causes the raised pustules characteristic of a herpes attack. Thus is demonstrated both latency and the presence of ineffective antibodies.

Not so, says Duesberg; these facts support my argument. He notes that the herpes virus shows latent and active periods – HIV is always latent. Furthermore, the level of antibodies increases as a herpes attack occurs, the antibodies contain the attack, and the antibody level falls. In AIDS patients the level of antibodies against HIV remains constant from its latent to its alleged 'active' phase. Far from suggesting by this example that HIV is a dangerous virus, sometimes latent and sometimes active and not controlled by antibodies, the herpes model suggests the opposite.

Some ninety per cent of AIDS patients tested for antibodies to HIV are antibody-positive. This is not dissimilar to the figures for antibodies to Esptein-Barr and cytalomegalo viruses which are also found in AIDS patients. Antibodies to hepatitis B are also present in ninety per cent of drug addicts who are HIV antibody-positive.

Why should there be people who have AIDS but do not have the antibody to the virus? Duesberg would say, of course, it is because the virus doesn't cause AIDS and there could easily be one hundred per cent of AIDS patients without the virus. If we can have one patient without the virus, then obviously it is not necessary for the disease.

The supporters of the HIV hypothesis also have to deal with this question. Paul Feorino from the Centers for Disease Control said:

> We don't get one hundred per cent antibodies to HIV in frank AIDS cases because our results aren't good enough. Our tests won't pick up all the antibody positives.
>
> When people are in the last stages of AIDS of course they aren't producing antibodies to anything, their immune systems have completely given up. Early in the infection they won't show up seropositive, there's a 'window' period between infection and developing antibodies. Some people just don't create antibodies, their body doesn't produce them. We've been studying people since 1981 and I can definitely say HIV is a necessary element in AIDS.

Another paradox of the HIV hypothesis is that there are said to be carriers of HIV who are at high or low risk of contracting the syndrome. This implies HIV is not sufficient to cause AIDS. As Duesberg said: 'Once they said that HIV alone causes AIDS. Now they say it's HIV plus co-factors. Well, if you say that AIDS is caused by HIV plus something else, until you know what the something else is, you are really only speculating about both of them as the cause.'

AIDS with no HIV

If HIV does not cause AIDS, wouldn't this have been apparent from HIV antibody-negative cases long ago? In fact, HIV positivity is often not used to diagnose AIDS, particularly in centres of the epidemic where the symptoms of AIDS are well-known and doctors feel no need to send off samples to laboratories.

In cases reported to the Centers for Disease Control from New York City and San Francisco, less than seven per cent have the result from an antibody test. In other areas the figure is much higher; in New Jersey sixty per cent of cases have had an antibody test, but one-third of US cases come from New York and San Francisco.

The CDC's original definition of AIDS was of a series of 'markers' of AIDS which indicated an underlying immune defect. These were infections caused by organisms which would not cause serious illness in a healthy body: Pneumocystis carinii; Cryptosporidium; herpes simplex; Candida albicans; cytomegalovirus; Toxoplasma gondii; Aspergillus; Cryptococcus neoformans; Nocardia; Strongyloides; atypical Mycobacterium; papovavirus. There are also four cancers: Kaposi's sarcoma; non-Hodgkin's lymphomas; Hodgkin's disease; Burkitt's lymphoma.

As may be imagined, the most easily visible signs were in fact the ones used – early cases were diagnosed on the basis of Kaposi's sarcoma or Pneumocystis carinii pneumonia.

In June 1985 the CDC revised its original criteria to make an official AIDS patient one who: tested positive for HIV antibody; had a low number of helper T cells or a low ratio of helper-to-suppressor T cells; widespread histoplasmosis (a fungal infection); isoporiasis causing chronic diarrhoea; candidiasis involving the lung; non-Hodgkin's lymphoma; Kaposi's sarcoma in patients no more than sixty years old.

This required an unacceptable level of lab work which discouraged doctors from reporting. They were there to treat the patient, after all, not to spend valuable time taking samples when they could tell from the Kaposi's lesions and the oral candidiasis that they had an AIDS patient.

Finally the CDC introduced a new definition of AIDS which came into effect on 1 September 1987. There are three sections which are related to the likelihood of physicians reporting with different standards of evidence rather than, as previously, setting a paradigm which doctors had to aim for.

Under the new criteria anyone who tested positive for HIV should be considered to have AIDS if they had, additionally, any of the specified indicator diseases, whether they were diagnosed by lab tests or by the physician's own experience.

If there were no evidence of HIV infection – either no test was done or the result was inconclusive – all that would be required would be a definitely diagnosed indicator disease with no other cause of immunodeficiency.

Most interestingly, when laboratory evidence is definitely against HIV being present – when the patient has tested HIV antibody-negative – the CDC is still prepared to accept a diagnosis of AIDS when there is either definitely diagnosed Pneumocystis carinii or both a specified disease definitely diagnosed and a low T helper count.

The new criteria increased the list of indicator diseases and also included, for the first time, the decline of the mental and motor faculties known as AIDS dementia. The frequent changes in the reporting criteria make it difficult to establish trends in patterns of AIDS cases and AIDS deaths, though it is obvious that a jump in figures immediately after the criteria change, out of keeping with previous figures, is a statistical artefact rather than a change in the pattern of the epidemic.

The revised definition of AIDS which came into effect on 1 September 1987 increased the number of reported cases in San Francisco by nineteen per cent in the last four months of 1987. It is not known how many of these were people who had previously shown negative for an HIV antibody test and were rejected for an AIDS definition. Under the new guidelines, it is worth repeating, AIDS patients are officially accepted as such even when their laboratory tests are negative for the presence of antibodies for HIV.

HIV with no AIDS

'It was said that ten to twenty per cent of the population of Haiti have HIV,' Peter Duesberg said, 'so there should be 100,000 AIDS deaths per year there, in a country of five million people and assuming a latency period of five years. In fact the incidence of AIDS is estimated at less than 0.01 per cent of the population.'

Even among high-risk groups, the incidence of AIDS seems to have no relationship to the incidence of HIV. In the US up to sixty-seven per cent of homosexual or bisexual men are antibody-positive, as are up to eighty-seven per cent of drug addicts and up to eighty-five per cent of haemophiliacs, yet the annual incidence of AIDS among these groups was found to average 0.3 per cent and to reach a peak value of 5 per cent in some locations.

In the population of the US as a whole, the estimate for years was of 1.5 or 2 million people infected with the virus. A White House report in 1987 found it to be an over-estimate and placed the figure at 680,000. The number of AIDS cases as a percentage of these infected individuals is still very small even with the reduced figures: in the first six months of 1988 10,380 cases were known. The highest number of deaths had occurred in the first six months of 1987 with 5582. So AIDS cases were 1.5 per cent of the lowest estimate of those infected and 0.5 per cent of the highest estimate. The cumulative number of AIDS cases in the US was 216 per million of the population. European rates are far lower, with the highest three countries being France 55.3, Switzerland 53.8 and Denmark 44.7 for the last six months of 1987. The figure for the UK was 21.6.

Evidence for the high level of HIV in the American population who are not at risk comes from various sources. John Beldekas talks of research by the State of Massachusetts into HIV in the blood of new-born babies. In the US a tiny amount of blood is taken from babies on an anonymous basis. In Massachusetts they tested it for HIV and found there was one to two per cent reactivity. It wouldn't have been remarkable to find this if there were a vast number of intravenous drug users in Boston, say, and if the blood samples all came from that area, but this was not the case. As he said: 'These were not just from one area, they were not the children of the poor, these cases were evenly spread out throughout the state. These babies were not born to people in quote "risk" groups, they were also born to white Protestant women. And yet you don't see a corresponding level of AIDS in the population – among the babies or the mothers.'

Another hint of the amount of HIV in the general population came when the US blood supply was screened in 1985. Almost 600,000 units of whole blood were screened. The total amount repeatedly HIV antibody-positive was a quarter of a per cent – over 1400 units. Unlike the donation of plasma, the donation of whole blood is voluntary (i.e. not paid for) in the US so these donations are not necessarily from high-risk groups but might well be representative of the most public-spirited of US citizens. As there are 12 million donations of blood, there could be, on these figures, 30,000 units of contaminated blood. This must have caused the Department of Health some concern because in March 1987 it was declared that all 30 million transfusion recipients between 1977 and 1985 were to be tested for HIV positivity.

Regardless of the vast statistical differences between those who have HIV and do not have AIDS, it is true that there is some coincidence between those who do have AIDS and those who have HIV. Duesberg said:

I think the reason why so many people of the risk groups are positive is because the virus is an indication, a marker, of promiscuity. This virus is available on the microbiological market – it's around but it's not endemic yet. You have to expose yourself to a great deal of intimate contacts, like a promiscuous homosexual or an intravenous drug user, then along with all the other infections you get, you will also pick up this virus.

AIDS patients have many viruses to a greater degree than the rest of the population. They are, like this one, markers of promiscuity. This also means they are very indirectly a marker of who might get AIDS because those who will get AIDS are from those groups.

The people who are at risk are those who are exposed to many things and the risk is extrapolated from them to the rest of the community. This is essentially like assessing the risk of driving a car by studying formula one drivers, race car drivers who go at 300 miles an hour and in a car that looks very different from the Chevvie that we drive across the Golden Gate Bridge at 55.

Duesberg's *Cancer Research* paper cites research among native male and female Indians of Venezuela where 3.3 per cent to 13.3 per cent have antibodies to HIV but none have symptoms of AIDS. The Indians are totally isolated from the rest of the country in which only one haemophiliac was reported to be virus-positive. Their having virus but no AIDS is thus unlikely to be a consequence of a recent introduction of the virus into their population.

The original researchers into this subject were criticised by HIV supporters who noted that malaria was endemic in this area and HIV tests can give a 'false positive' result: misinterpreting malaria antibodies for HIV antibodies. Leaving aside the implications this revelation has for the vast estimates of HIV infection in equatorial Africa, the point surely is that either you do have faith in a test or you don't. These Indians were tested three times by the three different tests which are claimed to be foolproof methods of detecting HIV when used in the US and Europe. But when the tests don't back the theory, it must be the tests which are wrong, not the theory. To add to the evidence in the Venezuelan Indian story – tribes in a similar position in neighbouring Brazil were tested and found to be HIV antibody-negative by the same tests even though malaria of the same type as that which affects the Venezuelans is also endemic in their area.

Yet another retrovirus was later recruited to account for the discrepancy. It was the latent South American Retrovirus (SA-RV). Of course this is a perfectly adequate explanation of why antibodies against a retrovirus were found in the Venezuelans. They did have a retrovirus, it just wasn't HIV. In only a decade of studying them it has become apparent that latent retroviruses are extremely common. The real question about this explanation is why it is used only to support the

HIV hypothesis when it falls down. How many of those who are AIDS patients or HIV antibody-positives are classified as such because their 'AIDS test' reacted to an exotic retrovirus which was not HIV? How about the West American Retrovirus or the East American Retrovirus? They are probably there if we look for them and are probably responsible for a whole cohort of false positive tests.

How can a supporter of the HIV hypothesis like Abraham Karpas account for the vast discrepancy between those with HIV infection and those with AIDS? He said:

> You can ask with any infection why isn't everyone developing the disease. Fortunately we have – most of us have – a very efficient immune system which develops antibodies to micro-organisms including AIDS and protects us from becoming ill.
>
> However, AIDS is probably one of the most deadly viruses around. It may be as high as twenty-five per cent of individuals who have the virus will develop AIDS but it will take nearly twenty more years before we know the percentage of those infected who come down with the disease.

A dormant retrovirus

Central to Duesberg's assault on the HIV hypothesis is his argument about the nature of the virus itself. Over twenty years of studying viruses has taught him a great deal about their nature. He says a retrovirus like HIV could not, by its nature, kill cells. It has to live in peace with its host.

Indeed, far from killing cells, retroviruses often stimulate their growth. It was for this reason that they were considered the most plausible viral causes of cancer – cancer being a disease of the proliferation of cells. AIDS, of course, is the opposite, a disease characterised by the decline in the number of T4 cells in the body.

This is radically different from the behaviour of 'cytocidal' or 'cell-killing' viruses. These viruses, whose behaviour has been studied for far longer than that of the retroviruses, will enter a human cell and use the material of the cell to replicate, almost as if they were feeding on it. Once the amount of virus in the cell has reached a critical point, the virus kills the cell. After it has died the virus particles or 'virions' swim cell-free in the blood looking for more cells to infect.

A retrovirus, by contrast, will rely on a living and dividing host for its replication. The retrovirus builds itself into the cell's reproductive system.

Cells reproduce by mitosis – each part of the cell divides in two so there are now two cells where previously there was one. When this happens to a cell carrying a retrovirus, the retrovirus too, as it has become part of the genetic makeup of the cell, reproduces by mitosis. The cell has duplicated its parasite along with itself.

It is this reliance on its host which makes the retrovirus so benign, Duesberg says. 'Retroviruses, in particular at low titres, are unlikely to be the cause of any disease, including AIDS. In fact, they are so benign that many retroviruses have become part of what's called the "germ line", the regular chromosomes of healthy animals. That includes mice and chickens which contain fifty to a hundred retroviruses which have the same genetic makeup as HIV. They are not the same, but they have the same genetic structure.'

Duesberg considers that HIV simply doesn't do enough to be a virus causing a deadly disease, it is biochemically inactive. Once it has entered a cell, it simply stays there duplicating along with it. He says:

In order to cause a disease you have to do something, you have to make DNA, you have to make RNA, you have to make protein. You have to make some toxin, have to invade a significant percentage of your target cells. This virus doesn't do that at any stage of the disease.

This virus is dormant all the time, it never becomes active. We are being told it's dormant to begin with, it's dormant when you suffer from it, it's dormant when you die from it. There is no report in the literature describing the virus ever to be active in a patient, only in cell culture.

There is no parasite that I know of among viruses and bacteria and fungi that is dormant when it is pathogenic. This one is supposed to be. This is one of the main reasons why I don't believe that this virus is the cause of AIDS.

In Africa, everybody or at least most people have leprosy bacillus, but very few have leprosy. When they do have it, or when we have tuberculosis or herpes blisters, then these microbes become locally or systemically active. The 'AIDS virus' continues to be dormant even when patients are dying from AIDS.

Duesberg's complaint about the alleged long latency period of HIV is supported by the discrepancy between the long latency period of AIDS and the short life cycle of HIV.

Infection with HIV produces a mononucleosis (glandular fever-type) illness one to eight weeks later. The infection lasts one to two weeks, until anti-viral immunity is established – the B cells start producing HIV antibody, making the person 'antibody-positive'.

By contrast, the time lag between infection and the appearance of AIDS is estimated from transfusion-associated AIDS to be two to seven years. The average latent period was estimated to be five years in adults.

But helper T cells duplicate themselves around once every thirty days – and if they are carrying a retrovirus they duplicate that too. Duesberg wrote in *Cancer Research*: 'In view of the claim that the virus directly kills T cells and requires five years to cause disease, we are faced with two bizarre options: either five-year-old T cells die five years after infection or the offspring of the originally infected T cells die in their fiftieth generation.'

In other words: supporters of the HIV hypothesis must either believe that infected T cells will stay alive for perhaps sixty times their natural lifespan and then suddenly be killed by their retrovirus parasite, or they must believe HIV will peacefully co-exist and divide with the T cell fifty or sixty times and then decide to kill it.

If HIV were really a killer virus, the most obvious thing for it to do would be to kill soon after infection – before the body had built up anti-viral immunity.

There is one other possibility – that HIV carries with it a 'time bomb' gene which will make a harmless passenger virus pathogenic after a certain period or when some other event occurs in the body. A great deal is known about retroviruses and one of the things which is known is the genetic structure of the organisms – they need all their genes to replicate, there are none left over which might perform this function of a 'time bomb' or transforming gene.

It has been noted that HIV has two extra genes. Montagnier refers to them as Q and F genes, in addition to *gag*, *pol* and *env* which all retroviruses share. Could not these genes be the missing killers which Duesberg insists should be present if HIV causes AIDS? He explained that by a process termed 'deletion analysis' it was possible to tell that the extra bits of genetic material, even though we do not know what they do exactly, could not have a function other than reproduction.

In deletion analysis, genes are removed and the virus is studied to see what it *doesn't* do without the missing gene. Therefore it is possible to tell what the missing gene does. Duesberg said:

> You take the cloned virus and knock the gene out and see how the virus lives without it. The answer with all of these genes is that it doesn't. That's why I don't get excited about whether there are eight, nine or ten of them because, when you take them out, the virus doesn't grow any more so they must be essential for replication.
>
> You can analyse further and further, slice the salami thinner and

thinner, but though this is important for virology, it doesn't explain how that virus is said to kill. There are no genes to be spared, all are needed for replication.

Koch's postulates

Robert Koch was truly one of the pioneers of medicine who mapped out territory where previously only single travellers had ventured. Born in Klausthal, Germany, he was a doctor in various small towns, then a field surgeon during the Franco-Prussian war. It was when he became district surgeon in Wollstein that he was able to set up his own small laboratory, first studying algae.

Steps had been taken in bacteriology by Friedrich Henle, who theorised in 1840 that micro-organisms caused infectious diseases, and by Casimir-Joseph Davaine who identified microscopic rod-shaped objects in the blood of dead sheep as the possible cause of anthrax.

Koch had moved from studying algae to this new area of research. He cultivated the anthrax organisms and discovered the growth within them of oval bodies – dormant spores. These spores lie in pastureland for years until the right conditions make them develop into the rod-shaped organisms which cause anthrax.

This was the first time the life cycle of a bacteria had been described and the first time proof of the causal relationship between a micro-organism and a disease was possible.

Koch contributed considerably to the development of techniques for growing bacteria in culture media and for fixing them and staining them under a microscope.

His greatest achievement was the isolation in 1882 of the tubercle bacillus responsible for the scourge of tuberculosis. When an epidemic of cholera struck Egypt there were fears it would spread to Europe and Koch was sent as part of a German government commission to investigate the disease. In studies there and in India, after the Egyptian epidemic had subsided, he discovered the cholera organism and its transmission routes via contaminated water and infected clothing.

Koch's other work included discovering the cause of amoebic dysentery and a study of a wide range of diseases of man and other animals. He was awarded the Nobel Prize in 1905 for his tuberculosis work.

This sort of textbook biography (the above was derived from the *Encyclopaedia Britannica*) implies that the life of someone like Koch and the progress of medicine is a straight line: simply hunting down one microbe after another, identifying it, staining it and declaring it to be the cause of an illness. Next, please.

In fact, as usual, life was a good deal more complicated when it was actually being lived than it appears to be now when we read about the most important dates and events in the history books. We now know what mattered and what did not in the history of medicine. In the cacophony of theories and treatments of the past we pick out the voices which persisted through to the present day – theories proved correct by later discoveries, treatments whose use continued or were steps on the road to the treatments of today.

The past, of course, looked very like the present to the people who were living then. As medical writer James Le Fanu comments on the period after Koch's isolation of the tubercle bacillus:

> The 'germ theory' of disease was in the ascendant and the centuries-long belief that had attributed illness to the 'miasma' or the 'humours' was swept away. Very soon a specific germ or bacteria was being sought as the cause of each and every illness, and amidst all the enthusiasm error became inevitable: staining techniques can be faulty, smudges down the microscope can be deceptive and the human mind has a powerful influence over what the eye perceives. In particular, 'bacteria' were alleged to cause many diseases that we now know to be due to vitamin deficiency.

This is putting it mildly. What happened was that talented and well-equipped scientists took samples from their subjects, isolated micro-organisms, developed media in which to culture them, stained them and stared at them for long hours and declared them to be the cause of this or that disease, secure in the knowledge that they were making a significant contribution to human health and their own fame.

Le Fanu cites some of those who discovered the bacterium which causes beriberi:

> Glockner identified an amoeba, Fhaardo a haematozoan, Pereira a spherical micro-organism, Durham a looped streptococcus, Taylor a spirillum, Winkler a staphylococcus and Dangerfield an aerobic micrococcus. Christian Eijkmann was sent to Java by the Dutch government with specific instructions to find the bacterium responsible but fortunately disobeyed his masters and found it was caused by a deficiency of thiamine (a component of the vitamin B complex).

Into this hazardous world of conflicting claims and bacteria for all diseases, Robert Koch brought a set of principles. He worked out a series of rules to follow in order to determine whether a micro-organism actually causes a disease, the so-called Koch's postulates:

1. The organism must be found in all cases of the disease.
2. It must be isolated from the host and grown in culture.
3. It must reproduce the original disease when introduced into a susceptible host.
4. It must be found present in a host so infected.

In order to prove a disease is caused by a micro-organism it is necessary therefore to isolate the organism from a person with the disease, grow it under laboratory conditions, infect an experimental animal with it and then recover that same micro-organism from the animal.

How does HIV fare on this test?

HIV is not found in all AIDS patients, even if the antibody test, the test for activity against the virus, rather than the virus itself, is used.

The virus itself can be found in fifty per cent of antibody-positive people. It is present in small quantities – it is infecting one out of 10,000 or 100,000 cells but it is there.

Once isolated, it can be grown in culture, a considerable achievement of bench-work science. By this method millions of potentially infected cells are grown in cell culture, away from the suppressive immune system of the host, until free virus is detectable.

While it does not specifically relate to the second postulate, it is as well to mention what happens to HIV in cell culture. The cells where the HIV is being cultured die after fusing together – something they have never been claimed to do in an AIDS patient, though the death of cells in culture with HIV is often erroneously referred to as evidence that HIV kills cells.

This cell death happens fast, within a couple of weeks as opposed to the claimed five-year latency period in patients. It also only happens in the presence of very large amounts of virus, levels which are never seen in patients.

Essentially what occurs is that the surface of infected cells, studded with high quantities of virus, hooks on to the surface receptors of uninfected cells. Then an infected cell fuses with an uninfected cell by the same mechanism that otherwise fuses a free virus particle with an uninfected cell. When this happens often enough, there is a 'clump' of cells.

As for the third and fourth postulates: there is no animal model which could show HIV as causing AIDS. This of course could be because HIV does not cause AIDS. This is hardly a substantive argument as many human problems are notoriously difficult to reproduce in laboratory animals. All we can be sure of in this connection is that when chimpanzees are infected with HIV they develop a mononucleosis (glandular fever)-like illness which is transient and which declines as antibodies against HIV build up. Thereafter no problems.

A retrovirus which is similar to HIV has been found in African green monkeys but it does not cause a disease in them. It may well be that this virus can be considered a model for HIV though only within the species which is its host. Like HIV in humans, the monkey virus is not pathogenic, but is just a harmless traveller.

The last two of the postulates are confounded by the absence of an animal model but of course there are several million humans who have been inoculated with HIV with so little effect they are unaware it has happened. If a significant proportion were to go down with AIDS this would make it likely that HIV is the cause. It is likely, however, that those who support the HIV hypothesis will simply continue to extend the latency period – from five to ten to twenty years – the virus *will* cause AIDS, they will tell us, if only we wait long enough for it. Koch did not take this approach in account when he formulated the postulates.

To be fair to the retrovirologists, it is rather difficult in the days of machines which can detect one gene in 10 million to expect them to abide by the postulates which were formulated when pathogens had to be seen on a microscope slide or in a culture to be believed. Koch may have had problems isolating the tubercle bacillus from patients with tuberculosis. With modern techniques, it is possible to isolate the bacillus from almost everyone, and very few of them have the disease. Many of us have picked up this bacteria but our immune systems keep it in check, we will not develop TB.

The problem, Duesberg notes, is that biochemical thinking has not kept up with biochemical technology. He helpfully suggests three principles which could be used today to tell whether a micro-organism was a dangerous pathogen, actively damaging the host, or a passenger, whether potentially dangerous or not. His criteria for determining whether a micro-organism is pathogenic are:

1. It must be biochemically active. It must be doing something.
2. It must infect more cells than the host can spare or regenerate during the course of the infection. If it only damages 'spare' cells, there will be no problem apparent to the host.
3. The host must be permissive – it cannot suffer a damaging infection if it is immune to the infection, if it has functioning antibodies to it.

HIV fulfils only about one and a half of Koch's four postulates when it is challenged as the cause of AIDS. It does not fulfil any of Duesberg's criteria.

The dog that didn't

Duesberg uses as an epigraph to his *Cancer Research* paper a quote from Sir Arthur Conan Doyle's *The Sign of Four*: 'How often have I said to you, that when you have eliminated the impossible, whatever remains, however improbable, must be the truth.'

In this context the improbable is that scientists ran off after a passenger virus, simply because it was new and was present in many AIDS patients. The impossible is that it could cause a disease as serious as AIDS. It is latent, it is present in quantities which are too low and it does not have the necessary genetic information to do so. Duesberg has spent many years mapping the genes and genetic elements of animal retroviruses; it would be difficult to fault him on the genetic structure of a virus.

Another quote from Conan Doyle comes to mind in view of the reception the *Cancer Research* paper received:

'"Is there any other point to which you would wish to draw my attention?"

"To the curious incident of the dog in the night-time."

"The dog did nothing in the night-time."

"That was the curious incident," remarked Sherlock Holmes.'

Howls of protest might have been expected to greet Duesberg's paper. Letters should have come flooding in damning him and all his works in the most scientifically elegant manner. Experts in the various disciplines Duesberg touches on – retrovirology, genetics, epidemiology – should have written biting articles in reply, re-establishing the facts they knew so well. The AIDS establishment should have defended its corner.

In fact nothing at all happened. No one replied. Not even a letter. The editor of *Cancer Research*, Peter Magee, confirmed to me in January 1988 that none had been received and none was awaiting publication. 'Peter Duesberg is a distinguished scientist,' he said, 'he is a member of the National Academy of Sciences. I knew he had these views so I asked him to contribute. There was no response at all. I was surprised, I would have thought someone like Duesberg would have elicited a response from all the big names. I would have thought people involved in retrovirology would have leapt upon it.'

Duesberg said:

Supporters of the HIV hypothesis talk to reporters about how terrible it is what I've done when they are called up about it but nobody wants to reply.

I'm convinced now they don't have the answers. They have made all the claims and the vested interests are so great they can't go back now.

I have never seen a situation like this before. I know all the people involved here, I have known them fifteen or twenty years. We have been in the same retrovirus club. When there was a challenge to anyone's hypothesis they would strike back right away if they could. If they couldn't, they had lost the argument.

Of all the suspicious events surrounding the announcement of HIV as the cause of AIDS, the most suspicious is the one which did not happen – why were the academic dogs silent?

What would prove Duesberg wrong?

Peter Duesberg says HIV does not have any of the qualifications required for a disease-causing micro-organism: it is not active, it does not kill more host cells than can be replaced by the host's natural regeneration process and the host is protected from it by an antibody mechanism. Merely adding up arguments against HIV does not prove the case – though in any other scientific debate the HIV proponents would already have lost by default because of their refusal to defend their corner.

It is valuable to know what would prove Duesberg wrong, or one can end up with a debate where the ground is constantly changing. Obviously a continuing disparity between the cases of HIV infection and the cases of AIDS would be in favour of Duesberg's argument, though as so few cases are tested even for HIV antibody this information will probably not be forthcoming. AIDS and HIV are considered so interlinked that tests are often neglected and often it is not known whether an AIDS patient has even come into contact with HIV.

Of course if Koch's postulates were fulfilled for HIV that would be the end of Duesberg's argument. It is unlikely this could occur now. No animal model has been found so the possibility of introducing HIV into a laboratory animal and seeing if it develops AIDS is remote. There is only one record of the many hundreds of health workers with 'needle stick' injuries having developed AIDS. The person was 'accidentally self-injected with several millilitres of blood from a hospitalised patient with AIDS while filling a vacuum collection tube'; that is, the worker was given a transfusion of infected blood. Anything in it could have caused the disease.

More to the point, a laboratory worker might suffer a stick injury with an experimental strain of pure HIV. This has once happened but the lab worker has not developed AIDS.

The AIDS babies might give a sign one way or the other to Duesberg's ideas. Of course they could be dying because of anything, including syphilis, passed on from their mothers who almost exclusively have been intravenous drug users. But at least researchers know where the baby has been and know all the factors currently acting on that baby. If they were to check the titre of the virus in the baby at birth and then frequently up to the point of death from AIDS, and if the viral titre rose as the AIDS became more severe, it would give a proof of HIV causing AIDS.

The development of HIV specific drugs or vaccines would be an indication of causation. Some person with absolute faith in the HIV hypothesis would have to take the vaccine against HIV and then undergo an inoculation of blood from an AIDS patient known to be carrying HIV. If they did not even develop lymphadenopathy, this would be a valuable proof.

Robert Gallo's reply

Though Robert Gallo, in common with other scientists of the AIDS establishment, chose not to reply in an academic paper to Duesberg, a New York rock magazine did manage to get the Gallo line. *Spin* magazine had printed an interview with Peter Duesberg in their January 1988 edition and wished to publish a response from Gallo. A reporter named Anthony Liversidge succeeded in obtaining Gallo's own laboratory telephone number and persisted in attempting to speak to him, though staff always put him off. One night Gallo himself picked up the telephone and through sheer journalistic skill Liversidge managed to keep him answering question after question on Duesberg's points. To be entirely fair to Gallo it would be desirable to reprint the entire article (Gallo has refused to talk with me about the challenge to HIV) but, copyright law being what it is, a few quotes must suffice to give a flavour of the interview.

In answer to the question about low levels of virus in HIV patients, Gallo said:

> Low levels? He does not know what he is talking about. He is quoting our data that the virus doesn't infect a number of cells. Cock and horse shit. Baloney. He misinterprets the experiments we published. The virus doesn't infect only a small number of cells. It infects a lot of cells. It is only expressed at one time in a small number of cells.
>
> Furthermore, hasn't Duesberg ever understood indirect mechanisms in cell killing? There are immune responses to the virus that destroy the proliferation of the T cell. That's crystal-clear now. It is not just a matter of the virus going in and killing the cell directly. Does that take a genius?

The response is, of course, that it is only when a virus is being expressed from cells that it can be considered to have any role in a disease process. The proposal that the virus is encouraging the body to attack itself (auto-immunity) is well worth study. No evidence has been forthcoming for it yet. Gallo commented that the evidence for transfusion-related AIDS proved the causal link with HIV, though of course his opponents would say, if there was HIV in that contaminated blood unit, what else was there? Syphilis, cytomegalo? An unidentified AIDS pathogen? He argued that Robert Koch never satisfied his own postulates and that the AIDS-like disease in monkeys means we do have an animal model.

On the question of how a latent virus can cause a serious disease he said: 'Peter Duesberg doesn't understand latency. He works with chicken viruses which cause cancer in two weeks. Do you think you get cancer in two weeks in nature? You know as a layperson when you smoke cigarettes you don't get cancer the next day. With HTLV-I, the leukaemia virus we discovered, you don't get cancer for twenty years. He doesn't understand latency, it takes time for retroviruses in nature to cause disease.'

So Gallo is defending one of his discoveries with reference to another. Lung cancer and smoking seems a curious parallel to draw when he is attempting to demonstrate the 'success' of an infection in causing a disease.

Gallo reiterated his belief that HIV alone causes AIDS with no co-factors such as other infections or predisposing aspects of lifestyle. He said: 'HIV would cause AIDS in Clark Kent, given the right dose and the right strain of the virus. Given the right dose and the right route of administration and the right time in someone's life. Alone and of itself. No doubt in my mind.'

Gallo maintaining a rigid position on this is interesting because many other members of the AIDS establishment have moved to the co-factor theory as the AIDS cases have not kept up with the numbers of people infected with HIV. They call HIV a 'necessary' element though not the only element. Tony Fauci of the National Institute for Allergy and Infectious Diseases said: 'There are co-factors but not to the extent that some people misconstrue some other unidentified virus as the real cause. HIV infects the body's T4 cells but a variety of factors can influence the course of the disease, i.e. genital ulceration which will allow infectivity or if the immune system is activated by another seemingly harmless virus.'

This is a far cry from Gallo's simile that getting HIV is like being hit by a truck and looking for co-factors is as foolish as asking the accident victim if there were co-factors or if he is hurt because of the truck.

The other main line of retreat from the view that in HIV we have the most deadly pathogen to hit humanity this century is the statement – completely true, of course – that no pathogen kills one hundred per cent. If it did, it would die out. Pathogens like to keep some hosts alive, to speak anthropomorphically, so they can be passed on and enjoy survival.

HIV is currently said to kill between twenty and thirty per cent of those infected. That is the World Health Organization figure. Gallo puts it at fifty per cent. As there is an increasing discrepancy between the numbers infected with HIV and the numbers with AIDS, the figure will drop. How low? Robin Weiss said to me, by way of example of the principle that not everyone with a pathogen gets a disease, that only one per cent of people with polio virus get polio. If we did get to that figure with HIV, or anywhere near it, it would not be moving the goalposts, it would be moving the pitch.

Moreover, in all other diseases the virus titre becomes active and rises in those who are not just infected but who are going to get the disease. Not so with HIV. Comparisons with other diseases should be prepared to go all the way and compare everything about the two diseases; the percentage infected with an alleged pathogen is not enough.

Duesberg's criticisms refused to go away and the lay press, though not the scientific press, kept up a steady trickle of interest. The dispute attracted the attention of Jim Warner, a senior policy adviser in the White House Office of Policy Development. He invited both Duesberg and Gallo to a meeting in Washington on 19 January 1988 to present their data for analysis. Duesberg consented willingly, Gallo refused. Warner said that when he wrote a memo on the questions surrounding HIV he quoted René Descartes: 'At least once in your life, insofar as it is possible, you should doubt all things.'

Scientists reacted with some disdain to the idea that a politician should take an interest in such matters. Science writers for the lay press, protective of their access to scientists and their small pool of specialist knowledge, reacted with horror. Science, after all, is supposed to be above politics. But as it is not, and never has been, it is interesting to recall the philosopher Paul Feyerabend's advice: 'Nor is political interference rejected. It may be needed to overcome the chauvinism of science that resists alternatives to the status quo.'

Five

Five Hs

THE PREVIOUS CHAPTERS have stated that HIV is probably not the cause of AIDS. It must stay in as a candidate for the cause. It has many adherents and their collective voice in favour of the HIV hypothesis is hardly negligible. An inquiring mind, however, will look elsewhere while keeping HIV in reserve. Where to look? The people with AIDS are, of course, the only certain reservoir of information which can make the AIDS story comprehensible. This chapter looks at the original four risk groups to see what they can tell us about AIDS. It then looks at the risk group which did not get AIDS.

Haemophiliacs

Alan Brownstein sat in his New York office on 12 July 1982 as a man who had problems but not insurmountable ones. As the Executive Director of the National Hemophilia Foundation he was the intermediary between America's 20,000 haemophiliacs and the powerful organisations which controlled the blood products which alone could keep them healthy. He had been working on a national agreement on the use of a test which might detect the presence of hepatitis in blood and thus save haemophiliacs from receiving blood products contaminated with the virus. But the test was not fully reliable and would cost more than the industry would bear willingly. This debate about the purity of Factor VIII, the blood product haemophiliacs use, had existed for the almost twenty years of use of Factor VIII. Slowly but surely Factor VIII was moving towards becoming a perfectly pure product.

Brownstein is a big, genial New Yorker, tough enough to do a hard job but humane enough to do it without making too many enemies. Nothing was likely to frighten him that summer afternoon when his secretary put through a call from Bruce Evatt of the Centers for Disease Control.

'I don't want you to be alarmed,' Evatt said, 'and it may mean nothing at all, but in the last seven or eight months we've been coming up with cases of immune dysfunction among haemophiliacs that might be AIDS.'

Brownstein didn't really know what AIDS was but he remembered an article from a magazine about 'the gay plague'. What did that have to do with him or with haemophilia?

'Could you enlarge on that, Bruce? What "immune dysfunction"?'

'One death in Miami, a fifty-five-year-old came down with pneumonia. The doctors didn't like the look of it so they ran some tests. It was Pneumocystis carinii pneumonia, they hadn't seen it before. They thought it was due to contamination of his Factor VIII.'

'I've never heard of that before. What are the other cases?'

'We flagged the pentamidine file, that's one of only two drugs used to treat Pneumocystis – and all supplies come from Europe to us at CDC, we send it to physicians requesting it. There were two more requests for pentamidine for use in haemophiliacs, last month and this month, in Ohio and Colorado.'

'How are they?'

'They're sick, they're very sick, almost certainly they're going to die.'

'Are you sure about your diagnosis?'

'We're sure they have immune dysfunction. As for the rest, we can't tell yet. The man who died had been treated with steroids, perhaps that suppressed his immune response. The others – we're pretty sure they're not homosexuals or drug addicts. In fact, we're very sure. Look, maybe it's not Factor VIII, maybe there's some other explanation. I just wanted to let you know so you hear it from me before you read it in the newspapers because we're publishing on this in four days.'

'Bruce, if something's happening related to blood products, you can bet it's going to hit the general public, haemophiliacs are an early warning system.'

'I know.'

When the call was over Alan Brownstein gathered together all the information he could find on AIDS and read it. None of it added up – homosexuals, curious opportunistic infections, drug addicts – what did these people have to do with haemophiliacs? Haemophiliacs are just males with a clotting disorder which makes it necessary for them to inject Factor VIII. Sometimes they do it as much as once a day, sometimes they only need Factor VIII once every few years – it depends on the severity of the haemophilia and their physical condition at the time. Apart from needing clotting factor to be artificially introduced into their blood, haemophiliacs lead normal lives. They have families and work and enjoy life or suffer life much as any other group of people. So why them, and why did it have to happen now, when everything was going so well?

Haemophilia – the past

The dark age of haemophilia must stretch back to prehistory but the first written references are in Jewish writings of the second century AD, where Rabbi Judah the Patriarch exempted the third son from being circumcised if the two elder brothers had died of bleeding after circumcision. There are subsequent Rabbinical references which refer to fatal bleeding after circumcision in brothers or in maternally related boy cousins.

There are scattered references to such bleeding disorders throughout history but it was not until the last decade of the eighteenth century and the first years of the nineteenth that the distinctive genetic nature of transmission came to be understood.

J. C. Otto in 1803 noted that although only males showed the symptoms, the disorder was transmitted by unaffected females to a proportion of their sons, the affected males being known as 'bleeders'. Otto, an American haemophiliac, traced his pedigree back to a woman named Smith who had settled near Plymouth, New Hampshire, around 1720-30. It was not until well into this century that it was recognised that men too could carry the defective gene for passing on haemophilia – haemophiliacs generally did not live long enough to reproduce.

Queen Victoria was the most famous carrier of haemophilia, her eighth child was Leopold, Duke of Albany. He died of cerebral haemorrhage at thirty-one. His daughter was a carrier, as were two of his sisters. Seven of Victoria's great-grandsons were haemophiliacs, including the most famous of all, the Tsarevich Alexis who played his small part in the downfall of the Romanov dynasty during the Russian Revolution of 1917. The Tsar's regime would have fallen regardless of his haemophiliac son, borne by Victoria's grand-daughter Alexandra, but the weakness of the royal house because of the boy's illness played a contributory role. The fact that there was only this sickly child to inherit the Romanov mantle necessarily weakened Nicholas II's hold in a reign which was already an anachronism in Europe. Rasputin's ability to hypnotise and thus relieve Alexis's pain gave this talented psychopath an influence over private affairs within the royal family and affairs of state.

In the first decades of this century haemophilia (meaning 'love of blood') came to be described in a recognisable form: it was known to become apparent clinically as excessive bleeding including internal bleeding; it affected males and not females; it recurred in families; the time it took for haemophiliac blood to clot was longer than for non-haemophiliac blood in laboratory tests.

It was laboratory work from now on – the properties of blood were beginning to be understood and in 1937 A. J. Patek and F. H. L. Taylor at Harvard found that a part of plasma, precipitated from it by dilution and mild acid, would normalise the clotting of haemophiliac blood. They called it 'anti-haemophiliac globulin' but it has been known by international agreement as Factor VIII since 1962.

The history of concentrates which could be used to treat patients began in 1964–5 with 'cryoprecipitate'; this comes from the blood serum of a small number of donors – perhaps six to twelve. There was a problem with this early product, useful though it was: clotting activity was provided but the precipitate was so crude and was used in such quantity that 'volume overload' occurred. The body's plumbing was taking the strain of all that additional matter.

This problem was solved in 1968–9 with the development of Factor VIII concentrate from the plasma of 2,500 to 10,000 donors. This was known as the 'golden age' or the 'age of liberation' for haemophiliacs. Not only was this an effective and freely available clotting factor, but advances in production methods meant it could be 'freeze dried', bottled and given to haemophiliacs to use in their own homes. They would take the bottle of yellowish flakes out of their refrigerator, reconstitute it with the addition of distilled water and inject it themselves. For over a decade haemophiliacs enjoyed close to normal lives for the first time in human history.

The AIDS bombshell

When AIDS hit the haemophiliac population of the US, it hit them hard. As Alan Brownstein said: 'We went through a period of denial. We didn't want to believe this was happening and we tried to prove it wasn't – that this wasn't AIDS, it was just the response of bodies bombarded with blood products until their immune system gives up. There was denial by patients, denial by their families, by physicians. The physicians felt, "We have not healed, we have killed our patients", it was a very, very rough period.'

The CDC reported five more cases of AIDS in haemophiliacs in December 1982 and transfusion cases had begun to show up. Blood as a medium for the putative agent which transmitted AIDS was still a proposition which was resisted, in particular by the powerful blood bankers.

Part of Alan Brownstein's response to the crisis was to participate in work on a survey of haemophilia deaths since the introduction of clotting factor concentrates in the late nineteen-sixties. He said: 'Yes, haemophiliacs were dying, but they had a high mortality rate before AIDS came along. Perhaps ordinary haemophilia deaths were being mis-diagnosed as AIDS and the haemophiliac population didn't have AIDS at all.'

The survey found that a dramatic decline in haemophiliac deaths had occurred between 1968 and 1979 – thirty-three per cent in deaths attributed to haemorrhage-related causes. There were six deaths reported annually over this period which could be related to AIDS – opportunistic infections, cancers and auto-immune disorders. But they weren't sufficiently closely related; they were 'unspecified connective tissue disorders' or 'myeloid leukaemias'. The report concluded that the deaths were not sufficiently suspicious to be attributable in retrospect to AIDS and that the increase in AIDS cases since 1982 could not be attributable to improved diagnosis and increased awareness.

Even as the survey continued, it was clear an epidemic was burning its way through the haemophiliac population. There was one clear retrospective diagnosis of AIDS in 1981, eight in 1982, thirteen in 1983 and thirty in the first ten months of 1984. One other finding pointed to Factor VIII: those who used more of it were more likely to develop AIDS. This dose relationship implied either that Factor VIII itself predisposed to immune dysfunction or that there was an infectious agent about and the more Factor VIII was injected, the more likely a haemophiliac was to encounter a contaminated batch.

With thousands of donors contributing to each batch, the danger of one donor contaminating the entire consignment is alarmingly high.

When the CDC met to discuss this question in January 1983 there were still many questions. There were insufficient numbers of AIDS victims among transfusion recipients and haemophiliacs to justify action, many people at the 'blood meeting' claimed. Others felt there was a major public health crisis in which the twelve million-pint-a-year US blood business might be the vehicle for spreading AIDS from a small number of risk groups to the general population.

As well as epidemiological caution and an understandable desire not to alarm the public before they could be certain, the CDC representatives were brought face to face with a major civil liberties issue: to eliminate risk they would have to screen donors, that would mean keeping out Haitians on the grounds of nationality and homosexuals on the grounds of sexual preference.

Homosexual organisations did decide, independently of any pressure, to discourage donation by homosexuals until the cause of AIDS was found. It did not discourage everyone. The story was told of a closet homosexual who was implicated in a transfusion-associated AIDS case and who was found to be the organiser of his company's blood drive. He felt obliged to donate.

The way in which those at the highest risk for AIDS came to donate into the plasma pool is a measure of the public-spiritedness of the gay community and a warning of how good intentions can lead to disaster.

Tens of thousands of units of plasma were collected from homosexual men in the late seventies and early eighties. They were taken for use in the preparation of a vaccine against hepatitis B. This virus is endemic in the homosexual community so when researchers wanted a community which had a high level of antibodies to hepatitis B in its plasma, the homosexuals were approached. The gay community's clubs, magazines and organisations pulled together in publicising the drive for plasma donation. Of course, the group of people who had the most hepatitis B were the most promiscuous; their plasma was most useful.

The plasma was drawn off and gamma globulin for making the vaccine was extracted. Gamma globulin has not been associated with any cases of AIDS so the agent for AIDS, whatever that is, is unlikely to be in the gamma globulin; it was in the other portion of plasma that was left after the gamma globulin was taken away. What happened to it? It was thrown back into the plasma pool to be made into Factor VIII and other blood products. It would have been a shame to waste it.

Blood politics

Alan Brownstein called the blood and plasma dealers together in January 1983 to ask them to adopt screening procedures to discourage donations from high-risk groups. The commercial sector, involved in plasma collection, complied. The not-for-profit sector, collecting whole blood, refused.

To understand this it is necessary to comprehend the complex politics of blood and profit in the US. Why was it the multi-national pharmaceutical companies who acted in a public-spirited way, not the organisations dedicated to good works?

The big companies: Bayer, Baxter Travenol, Rorer and Green Cross, own subsidiaries which buy and sell blood products in a business which brings in an annual revenue of more than $1.5 billion. As business people, it is advantageous for them to have a 20,000-strong cohort of 'customers' who will continue to use their products, perhaps for the rest of their lives. The plasma sum on the balance sheet looks healthy and is likely to remain so; it is an amount which is likely to remain constant and can thus be used into the future to offset the gigantic costs of pharmaceutical research which, if successful, brings immense profits. On the other hand, haemophiliac organisations like the National Hemophilia Foundation want to ensure a constant supply of Factor VIII. If they place too many demands on the producing companies or taint the corporate image with lawsuits or criticisms of the quality of the product, the pharmaceutical giants will just pull out. Factor VIII pays, but it doesn't pay that well. Haemophiliacs need the pharmaceutical industry more than the pharmaceutical industry needs haemophiliacs. The relationship is, however, one of mutual respect.

As soon as there were questions about whether Factor VIII was contaminated with the active agent for AIDS, haemophiliacs were administering less to themselves. For the first time in more than a decade Alan Brownstein was receiving reports of haemophiliacs suffering crippling joint pain – a symptom of the deep internal bleeding which Factor VIII will prevent.

The blood banks, on the other hand, have no such direct relationship with haemophiliacs and no special obligation to them. They collect whole blood and sell it to hospitals for whole blood transfusions. In this they compete against each other – the Red Cross is by far the biggest with revenues of $466 million a year. It does battle with the American Association of Blood Banks with 2,400 members, mostly hospitals and community blood centres, and with the Council of Community Blood Centers which represents regional blood banks. These may be known as not-for-profit organisations but this does not make their products cheap. 'Think of us as tax-exempt rather than not-for-profit,' said a leading figure in the AABB.

The blood products which the whole blood can be broken into – including Factor VIII – are sold along with the products the big companies obtain from plasmapheresis centres. As well as the advantage of not paying tax, the not-for-profit organisations do not have to pay their donors so they can enjoy a considerable commercial advantage over their rivals. Their main concern is the maintenance of their own viability and for this they must keep the voluntary donors coming.

They were concerned about the difficulties inherent in asking donors about their sex lives in order to exclude homosexuals. This might be considered invasion of privacy by homosexuals, it would be resented by non-homosexuals and, anyway, what is a homosexual? Does one homosexual experience make a person a homosexual? A recent homosexual experience? If transmission is sexual, there are few practices, if any, that two men can indulge in which cannot also be experienced by a man and a woman. If the transmission is through the use of recreational drugs, homosexuals are hardly the sole users of them.

The lack of knowledge about the cause of AIDS and its exact means of transmission was another reason for delay. A statement made to justify the blood banks' position said: 'Evidence that AIDS can be spread by blood components remains incomplete.'

There was also concern that public fear and ignorance would jeopardise the operation. The public might confuse giving infected blood with receiving it. Incredibly, the blood banks were correct and as recently as March 1987 a survey found that forty-two per cent of Americans believe AIDS can be contracted by giving blood. Other observers might have felt a public education programme was more in order than inaction put down to public ignorance.

The blood-donor screening decision betrayed a form of behaviour which is characteristic of the pattern of all dealings with AIDS since the epidemic became apparent. On the political, social and scientific fronts, the story was always the same: refusal to recognise that there was a problem; insistence that the problem was someone else's responsibility; action taken too late and in too small a measure.

Alan Brownstein said: 'Haemophiliacs serve as an early-warning system for the safety of the blood supply. The message we were trying to communicate at that meeting was that we were blinking a yellow warning about the blood supply, we didn't want the industry to wait for a red light to take action.'

The persons unlikely to share needles with drug addicts or to have sex with a promiscuous homosexual faced the danger of AIDS only through finding themselves in hospital, perhaps after a sudden accident, and requiring a blood transfusion.

The red light for the blood banks came in March 1983 when the US Public Health Service announced that high-risk groups shouldn't donate and the Food and Drug Administration issued donor-screening guidelines. In the two months of inactivity from the blood banks, more than 1.5 million units of blood were collected. It is not possible to tell how many units were contaminated.

There were always three alternatives for the protection of Factor VIII: screen the donors to prevent the AIDS agent entering the blood supply; test the blood supply for 'markers' for AIDS; treat Factor VIII itself to destroy the agent.

A test for an imbalance in T cells was used in some blood collecting centres from July 1983 but it was expensive and unreliable as a test for AIDS. A test for antibody to hepatitis B was possible as a surrogate test for AIDS – people who had hep B probably were at risk for AIDS, so excluding their blood would probably exclude AIDS-infected blood.

This never enjoyed great support because of its expense – it would cost $2.50 to $5 per unit to conduct the test and many who did not have AIDS or hepatitis (only antibodies to hep B) would be excluded, costing the blood banks a great deal of money.

The HIV antibody test became available in March 1985. It is another surrogate test but it is capable of picking up donations from high-risk individuals.

Heat-treating of Factor VIII has been in operation since 1985. In theory the condition of the donor was irrelevant in that the plasma could be purified and rendered safe regardless. This was the theory. In fact there were still AIDS cases, though a smaller number. There were two problems with heat treating: the absence of an animal model for AIDS meant no batch of Factor VIII could be tested after heat treating to see if it was pure. The only test was to give it to haemophiliacs and see if they got AIDS. The other problem was the cost – every hour of treatment and every degree of heat reduced the amount of Factor VIII and therefore reduced the profit a company could make by selling it.

Nevertheless, in the face of evidence that the heat treating used was insufficient to neutralise the AIDS agent, in February 1987 the plasma brokers increased by a half both the length of time and the temperature at which their Factor VIII was treated, to sixty-eight degrees for seventy-two hours.

Haemophiliacs and their families acted as humans will in times of crisis: some with courage, some with cowardice. It was sad for haemophiliacs to suffer from AIDS; they had, after all, used only a medical product prescribed by their doctors. It was particularly sad for children, the first generation of haemophiliacs to grow up with a normal childhood until the plague hunted them out. Those who were only HIV positive, who did not have the disease and might never have it, were persecuted and the haemophiliac children who showed no signs of any infection were shunned and accused, by some strange contortion of logic, of being homosexuals.

The wives and girlfriends of haemophiliacs also had to stake a claim to a piece of the moral territory. Alan Brownstein said: 'There is an array of responses among spouses. Some say it won't happen and I won't listen to your advice. Some say we're in love and if it happens it happens. Some are getting divorced. Planned marriages which seemed before all this to have been made in heaven have not occurred. There is denial, there is compliance with safe sex guidelines and there is abstention.'

Though none had died, in November 1987 there were fifteen cases of AIDS among spouses of haemophiliacs in the US.

British haemophiliacs

Charles Rizza, with a small grey beard and a warm smile, heads the Oxford Haemophilia Centre which compiles statistics on haemophilia in the UK and maintains liaison between clinicians at the eighty-four other haemophilia centres in the UK. He had the benefit of the US experience of AIDS, so when the first case was reported to him in January 1983 he was not alarmed. 'We knew something was going on in the States,' he said, 'and that whatever it was, was transmissible by blood and we knew we would get it soon. I was waiting for the telephone to ring to report the first case. The first death was in April 1983 and since then we've had a steady trickle of deaths. In the past four and a half years we've had reported sixty-six cases of AIDS and forty-six deaths.'

Dr Rizza is not excitable. He points out that AIDS deaths have now equalled deaths from cerebral haemorrhage, the most common cause of death among haemophiliacs in the previous five years. But while this is obviously distressing, as there are over 5000 haemophiliacs in the UK, the number of deaths is not suggestive of a plague of historic proportions.

He is also critical of the merchants of doom who delight in appearing on television and predicting the end of civilisation as we know it. 'If you can do nothing but stand up and promote pessimism then it's best to do nothing. It's completely counter-productive, it only upsets patients and you have more work to do calming patients as well as looking after them in other ways and you are no further forward.'

Families in Britain seem to have coped with AIDS in haemophiliacs more calmly than their American counterparts. As yet there are no AIDS cases among the wives of haemophiliacs and many people have continued to practice unprotected sex. Half a dozen healthy children have been born to the wives of haemophiliacs with HIV antibodies and no child of a haemophiliac has developed AIDS.

Early cases of AIDS in the UK could be put down to imported Factor VIII and the government was severely criticised for failing to complete the building of the Elstree fractionating plant which will make the nation self-sufficient in terms of the technology necessary to produce Factor VIII. Whether Britain can be self-sufficient in the plasma itself depends on the level of donations, which are all voluntary.

Despite all the concern about haemophiliac AIDS, HIV itself has never been isolated from Factor VIII. Perhaps this is because HIV is a sensitive virus and it is all but destroyed in the processing procedure for Factor VIII. It must have been present because patients developed antibodies to it but in Factor VIII itself the virus evades detection.

Many other viruses and other micro-organisms are similarly undetectable in Factor VIII – the pathogen which causes non-A non-B hepatitis, for example. The agent for this form of hepatitis is simply not known, it is only known that it exists in Factor VIII.

It will be remembered that on Robert Gallo's check-list of reasons why he thought AIDS was caused by a virus in the first place was the fact that: 'Factor VIII transfusions could transmit the agent and these materials are filtered in a way that should remove bacteria and fungi.'

The filtration method should remove bacteria and fungi and it does remove most of them, but some bacteria are small enough to get through the 0.22 micron filter which is used. There are other types of micro-organism, some of which come close to being bacteria and some of which come close to being viruses, which also get through, as well as the viruses themselves. The fact that the agent for AIDS is present in Factor VIII does not mean it has to be caused by a virus, though it does mean the larger bacteria, which would not get through the filter, are excluded as a causative agent.

Of course, if AIDS is caused by a virus, there is still the question of which virus. HIV is far from being the only one present in AIDS cases. Charles Rizza said:

> We recognised in the mid-seventies and early eighties that all of the concentrates were infected with non-A non-B hepatitis. The only way we knew was that when we had someone in who needed Factor VIII but who did not have hepatitis, we would transfuse him and he would invariably get hepatitis but not hepatitis-A or hepatitis-B. All we know is that there is that agent in the Factor VIII. The companies were going through a variety of tests to make the Factor VIII safe and they were halfway there when AIDS came along and presented a new problem. Factor VIII is still very impure, it could be called a crude protein concentrate contaminated with Factor VIII.

In the US it is estimated that as many as 19,000 severe illnesses or deaths may be annually attributed to non-A non-B hepatitis. It is less glamorous than AIDS for which there were 9784 deaths in 1986, the worst year of the epidemic, but it is still deadly.

Transglutaminase

Rising out of the trees of Long Island, New York, is a great black shape like a space ship on its launch pad. It is the State University of New York at Stony Brook and near the top is the Department of Urology where Richard Ablin is investigating a strong link between homosexuals and haemophiliacs.

Urology is that part of medicine which deals with the diseases and abnormalities of the urinary tract, though Richard Ablin is best known for his contribution to prostate gland surgery where he pioneered cryosurgical techniques: freezing the tissues during surgery. He thus spent a great deal of time looking up men's behinds.

Ablin, a big, lumbering, red-bearded bear of a man, had been studying the immunosuppressive effect of an enzyme called transglutaminase in the late seventies. He found transglutaminase in human semen and also in Factor VIII. This explained a mystery about haemophilia. He said: 'We wondered why asymptomatic, heterosexual haemophiliacs had immune profiles that were almost identical to patients with full-blown AIDS. We found through collaborative studies with two Hungarian doctors that we were able to identify in Factor VIII the same enzyme as in seminal plasma though with a different molecular form.'

He considers that the lining of the rectum is torn in anal sex, perhaps not seriously but sufficiently to allow seminal fluid, carrying transglutaminase, to come into contact with the cells of the immune system. Women would not suffer similarly through vaginal sex because the lining of the vagina is thicker and less likely to suffer trauma. Repeated anal sex in a woman might produce the same immunosuppressive condition. Haemophiliacs would be injecting the transglutaminase directly into their blood stream where it could interfere with the immune system.

The transglutaminase is believed to inhibit natural killer cells: those which destroy the body's own cells which have been infected with an outside organism.

Richard Ablin wrote to the *Lancet* in April 1985:

Association is not proof of cause, and agents such as (HIV) may turn out to be passengers on an already sinking ship. It would be reasonable to postulate some other transmissible agent, even a non-infectious one, which contributes to immune dysfunction and possibly predisposes to opportunistic infections. . . . As an alternative to the hypothesis that AIDS is solely an infectious disease I suggest that the opportunistic infections and tumours such as Kaposi's sarcoma seen in AIDS patients result from a combination of lifestyle hazard and immunodeficiency, whereas in patients with haemophilia the infections are a consequence of immunosuppression resulting from infusion of anti-haemophiliac factor.

This is not a complete answer to the question of the cause of AIDS. There is still the problem of transmission – the active homosexual partner developing AIDS, for example, though he had never received an inoculation of semen.

The pattern of AIDS strongly suggests a transmissible agent though the limited number of cases outside 'risk groups' argues for additional co-factors working with that agent or preparing the ground for it.

Ablin's work would, in any event, seem well worth pursuing but the research funding is being taken up by HIV. As he said: 'There is no money that's really available to investigate alternative causes of AIDS. We are told that research funds are available for AIDS research but when it actually comes to giving you the money, the funds aren't there. The virus or the viral etiology continues to be the emphasis. Tremendous amounts of money are being spent on developing vaccines against the virus. If the virus is not the causative agent of the disease, what good will a vaccine do?'

When I left Richard Ablin it was as I had found him: alone in a complex of offices and empty laboratories. The ELISA machine and the contamination hood were empty. No one had called while I was there. There was all the equipment for top-level research plus Ablin's first-class record in the field but unless he was prepared to look at HIV, there would be no money for staff. That has been another effect of the epidemic: to strip laboratories of creative work, all edged out by the ubiquitous HIV.

Haitians

Dominique was feeling unwell. The thirty-two-year-old taxi driver in Miami, Florida, was feeling dizzy and confused. He kept forgetting where he was driving and was unable to concentrate. He got the change wrong for his fares and had to ask passengers to tell him the way, even to easy locations. What was worse, persistent diarrhoea made it difficult for him to stay in his cab at all.

He went back to Jackson Memorial Hospital. He had been there six weeks before for treatment for his bad chest. He knew what that was, there had been enough coughing and spitting in the streets in Port-au-Prince for him to recognise tuberculosis when he had it. But this bout of TB didn't go away with antibiotics. It died down and came back with renewed virulence.

As he waited to see the doctor he pondered his fate. It was so miserable to have fallen sick just at this time when he had got a job with a cab company and was able to pay his brother back some of the money he had loaned when Dominique arrived, two years before, on an illegal boat from Haiti. They had escaped from the squalor of Port-au-Prince and, though poor in American terms and living in an overcrowded tenement, by comparison with the island they left, they were enjoying almost undreamt of luxury.

Dominique's English wasn't great, his first language was Creole and his second French, but when he had been examined and the doctor walked out of the door with her colleague he could swear he heard her say: 'It's another one of them.'

Haiti wasn't doing so well before AIDS; the epidemic was a death blow. Haiti is always described in statistics – eighty per cent illiteracy; fifty per cent infant mortality; average income of $250 a year; 10,000 political prisoners; one of the ten poorest countries in the world.

The island was discovered in 1492 by Christopher Columbus' sailors. There were a million native Indians and they were friendly. Perhaps they were too friendly. In forty years their numbers had dropped to 4000 – a consequence of an unprotected society being exposed to smallpox, scarlet fever, measles, yellow fever and, probably, the world-wide epidemic of the fourteen-nineties, syphilis.

The depleted population was made up from slaves from the West Coast of Africa. In French hands the colony became immensely wealthy, providing one-half of the revenues of the 'Sun King', Louis XIV.

Following the American and French revolutions, Haitians too fought and gained their freedom under the 'black Jacobin' Toussaint L'Ouverture. Their constitution proclaimed that Haiti would never be ruled by a white man as well as many fine egalitarian sentiments. As a Haitian proverb has it: Constitutions are made of paper, but bayonets are made of iron.

Haiti then suffered a series of dictators of almost comic awfulness, who busied themselves having impressive palaces built and thinking up grand titles for themselves. There were kings and emperors of Haiti and, in this century when emperors had somewhat fallen out of fashion, Dr François Duvalier had himself 'elected' President-for-Life.

Duvalier, known as 'Papa Doc', and his son Jean-Claude, known inevitably as 'Baby Doc', ruled Haiti for twenty-nine years with the sort of ruthlessness which gives dictators a bad name. Papa Doc set up a private army called the Tonton Macoute from the Creole words for bogeyman. Bad Creole children would be told Tonton Macoute, 'Uncle Knapsack', would come and carry them off in his sack. The Duvaliers built up this force of bogeymen until they outnumbered the regular army by two to one. They also kept an army of informers and people reliant on them for favours until the situation arrived where nothing could be achieved in Haiti except by members of the Tontons or people who paid them off. Their local autonomy in fact meant that even the Duvaliers had no control over them and were supported by the Tontons because they maintained the power structure which allowed the Tontons to function.

In a similar relationship to the dictators and also enjoying Duvalier patronage were the hougnans, the voodoo priests who kept the illiterate population under control with blood rites and zombification. Probably few people were zombified – drugged with an extract of puffer fish to make them appear dead. They could be brought round by the hougnan after burial and exhumation to be placed in a hypnotic trance in which condition they would do the hougnan's bidding. The point is not that they created a nation of zombies but that by creating a few they struck the rest of the 5 million population in fear for their souls.

Paradoxically, Haiti is a Catholic country, though the Haitians seem happy to combine voodoo with Christianity – Papa Doc proclaimed himself Baron Samedi, the devil who rose on the Saturday between Good Friday and Easter Sunday.

A tiny percentage of Haitians, just a few thousand, enjoyed a lifestyle which would be considered luxurious even in wealthy countries. In general these would be educated, French-speaking Catholic mulattos. The vast majority of the population, illiterate, Creole-speaking voodoo-practising negroes, suffered extremes of poverty which can only be compared to the poorest African countries. In the nineteen-eighties life became worse even for these subsistence farmers. A prolonged drought lowered agricultural production on land which had already been declining in fertility because of over-intensive use.

Duvalier was said to survive on terror, voodoo and American aid. Some $54 million was given to Haiti in 1986, much of it being eaten away in graft to keep the regime in power.

With the decline in agriculture and the running down of the exhausted bauxite mines, Haiti had just one industry which was still thriving: tourism. The tourists generally were not going to visit the historic sites of Haiti – there weren't so many of those. David Black describes Haiti before AIDS in *The Plague Years*:

> On the main road from the Carrefour to the centre of Port-au-Prince are the big whorehouses, like the Club Social Cabaret, which are surrounded by massive walls. Inside are compounds with bars, shady groves and little hovels that the boys and girls use. In these 'social clubs', for the price of a blow-job in Manhattan, $25 to $50, you can do virtually anything with virtually anyone; male and female, children and crones.
>
> Such freedom offers not a test of sexual prowess but of the imagination. What do you want? A thimble-job, an around-the-world, the rear-admiral, the python dance, a rum-desire, the Macao Sling – which involves two chickens and some piano wire.

Heterosexual and homosexual sex tourists flocked to Haiti, 70,000 in the winter of 1981–2. Long before AIDS, Haitians were unhappy about medical publications showing an extremely high rate of syphilis among them.

The first AIDS cases were more of a puzzle than a cause for alarm to the doctors at Jackson Memorial when they first started presenting in 1981. There are around half a million Haitians in the US, many of them illegal immigrants. It was the most recent arrivals, the 'boat people', who were seen at the Miami hospital. A steady stream of them had been seen in recent years – all undernourished and tuberculous. Haitian AIDS patients had a particularly virulent form of TB; salmonellosis, giardiasis and other gut parasites leading to diarrhoea and under-nutrition; Candida albicans in the mouth and throat; Pneumocystis carinii which is normally associated with malnutrition (in the absence of AIDS); and the 'cat disease' Toxoplasma gondii. This infection, almost certainly an activation of a latent parasite, is far more common in Haitians than in non-Haitian AIDS patients, probably because Haitian culture would bring people into contact with animals far more than in industrialised societies. Haitian Americans tended not to have external Kaposi's sarcoma lesions.

It was 'toxo' which made doctors at Jackson Memorial most suspicious but until a CDC official telephoned in summer 1981, they simply treated the condition and the patients recovered. In fact, as is always the case with AIDS, aggressive treatment for one condition relieves that condition but the patient then succumbs to another opportunistic infection, then another.

The CDC investigator wanted to know if the hospital had seen any homosexual men with an immunosuppressive syndrome who were highly infected with cytomegalovirus. 'Well we don't have anything like that,' said George Hensley, who did the pathological examinations on Haitian brain tissue, 'but we do have several Haitians who've died with toxo and CMV in their brains.'

The response of the CDC man has not been recorded for posterity, presumably it was a request to repeat the information followed by an audible intake of breath.

It soon became clear, from checking hospitals in areas where there was a considerable Haitian settlement, that there were a great many Haitian AIDS patients – thirty-four recorded in summer 1982, more than 110 in summer 1983, with the Haitian Minister of Health reporting 157 cases in the island – almost certainly an underestimate because of the high death rate already prevailing and the lack of people able to diagnose the condition. Haitians with AIDS ranged from those who had only just emigrated to the US to those who had been resident for up to eleven years.

How did AIDS get to Haiti? It is claimed that Haitians had close contact with the Belgian Congo (Zaire) and Haitians took over professional and middle-management positions in Zaire when it became independent in June 1960. Belgian policy had been to restrict professional jobs to whites, so there were insufficient numbers of trained Africans to do them. Zaire was incubating the AIDS agent and it was passed on to Haitians during their sexual relations with the people of Zaire at some time over the next twenty years. This theory falls foul of the fact that AIDS was not present in Africa until around the same time it became apparent in the US – it might have been, and been misdiagnosed, of course, but it was not present in an endemic form.

This theory says the Africans gave AIDS to the Haitians who gave it to the homosexuals on sex holidays in Port-au-Prince who took it back to the US and infected the blood banks. While many people believe this theory, it is in fact based on as much fact as the theory that AIDS was a result of misguided lab research. It is just as likely that the homosexuals and others who went on sex holidays took the agent for AIDS to Haiti as that it happened the other way round. Indeed, Haitian authorities insist that this is just what happened but then, they would, wouldn't they, just as the establishment in the West would like to blame the despised minorities: black people, illegal immigrants, homosexuals. The truth, probably, is that we will never know where the agent which causes AIDS came from.

How did the Haitians transmit it, once some infectious agent had entered their population? This was the real mystery and one which would continue to perplex were it not for political manoeuvrings which have buried Haitian AIDS data amid a mass of other 'risk groups'.

From 1981, when it was clear there were Haitian cases of AIDS, the Haitians had been placed in a 'risk category', forming one of the so-called 4H Club of haemophiliacs, heroin users, Haitians and homosexuals. But what was the risk to Haitians?

They didn't receive transfusions and they were too poor to afford the hard drugs or even the syringes for drug addiction. Drug use might have accounted for some of the cases among Haitian Americans but it is unlikely that the doctors treating them would have overlooked signs of intravenous drug use, even if the patients had been denying it. They were also emphatically not homosexual. Homosexuality is a social crime in Haiti and goes against the macho image of Latin men – some Americans developed an aggressively masculine form of homosexuality but this was alien to Haitian thinking.

There were other theories – that voodoo practices using blood had spread the disease; that 'injectionists' giving a series of injections of a quack remedy with the same needle had done it; that knives used for ritual scarring on several people had transmitted it the same way.

None of these theories was satisfactory. When patients themselves were questioned they denied these practices but, then, they had denied homosexuality.

People who knew Haiti were convinced that the Haitian AIDS cases were homosexual, that they had been homosexual prostitutes but had not admitted to this when questioned partly because it wasn't their 'real' sexuality, but only something they had done for money; and partly because of the shame attached to homosexual practices.

As Jeffrey Vieira, Chief of the Infectious Diseases Service at the Brooklyn Hospital said: 'In the United States, despite concerted efforts to elicit histories of homosexuality, fewer than five per cent of Haitians will admit to such relationships at any time during their lives. Having distanced themselves from the poverty that promoted homosexual prostitution, and having assumed a more conventional lifestyle in the United States, most are understandably reluctant to make such admissions.'

Sheldon H. Landesman, Director of the Haitian AIDS Study Group at Downstate Medical Center, New York, told a conference in spring 1983: 'We are left with an epidemiological void in trying to explain how the disease is spread within the Haitian population. Neither homosexual practices nor blood appear to account for the disease within this population group. Attempts to accumulate the data that can explain the disease in this population are hampered by cultural and language barriers. Further difficulties may be encountered when trying to cross governmental and bureaucratic barriers.'

Honest doubt looks good on paper but it isn't much of a bargaining counter in the world of politics. The Haitian AIDS cases were about to demonstrate yet again that the bulldog of scientific inquiry rolls over to have its tummy tickled when the political paymasters snap their fingers.

Having an entire racial group stigmatised as disease carriers was one of the early horrors of the AIDS story. Homosexual men might conceal their sexual preference; heroin users could, with some difficulty, conceal their habit; haemophiliacs need tell no one of their condition. How could the black people who spoke with a French accent be hidden? Haitians lost their jobs, their children were discriminated against, they were shunned by other Americans. The announcement that high-risk groups shouldn't give blood seemed to confer an official seal of approval on blatant discrimination.

The indefatigable Ary Bordes, Haitian Minister of Health, was outspoken: 'The reluctance of Haitians to admit that they are homo-sexual or drug abusers, is responsible for their erroneous placement on the list of high risk groups for AIDS,' he said.

In a world increasingly hostile to America, particularly under the disastrous Reagan foreign policy, America needed all the friends she could get. The US might be rich and powerful but the world could get very lonely when the international community was slamming the doors behind them one by one. Haiti should be placated – it would be one problem fewer and what difference did it make? All it required was a change in the statistics. The CDC finally agreed, not without resentment, to re-allocate all the Haitian figures. There was no Haitian risk category, just admitted homosexuals and 'undetermined'.

Too late, though, to save the regime. The tourist trade collapsed. In two years Haiti changed from a swinging international resort into what it really was – a miserable backward country run by a corrupt dictatorship.

With unemployment at sixty per cent and no hope of economic recovery the Haitians had nothing to lose. Daily anti-government riots were not slowed by the Tonton Macoutes firing point-blank into crowds of demonstrators or, one of their favoured tricks, deliberately killing entirely innocent people in an attempt to strike terror into all hearts. The government declared a state of siege, the radio stations were closed, there were more arrests, beatings, shootings. False reports that Duvalier had fled the country were greeted with rejoicing then despair as the Macoutes asserted themselves. The army held back, knowing they would be the ones to take over after the people had won their freedom.

Finally, on 7 February 1986, President-for-Life Jean-Claude Duvalier, his wife Michele, two truckloads of luggage and around fifty retainers flew out of Port-au-Prince in a US Air Force C-141 transport jet. The AIDS epidemic had claimed its first coup. There was wild celebration but Haiti's problems were not yet over. The military authorities arranged free elections for December 1987 only to see them broken up by the Tonton Macoutes who had been too powerful to destroy in the retributions which followed the fall of Duvalier.

One need not be too cynical about the politically expedient alteration of the AIDS figures. It is perfectly possible that the Haitian Minister of Health was correct and existing risk factors could account for Haitian AIDS with no reference to nationality being necessary.

Haitians, after all, had the indicators of other risk groups: high levels of cytomegalovirus, herpes simplex, Epstein-Barr virus, hepatitis A and B. It is quite possible they were picked up through prostitution. The high number of women AIDS patients in Haiti could be accounted for by the fact that anal sex is a frequent practice in countries like Haiti where contraception is too expensive to obtain. Additionally, the men who were only part-time prostitutes would also have wives and girl-friends and they would practice a good deal more heterosexual sex than 'real' homosexuals would, so the spread to women was more likely.

Even given all that, it is hard to ignore the quality data presented in leading medical journals by people who set out to look into this question. In the 20 October 1983 *New England Journal of Medicine*, the most intensive study which could be conducted into the lifestyle of Haitian AIDS patients was published. It was a collaborative effort between US and Haitian researchers. Sixty-one patients were questioned in their own language by physicians who knew local customs. The number who could be persuaded to admit to homosexual encounters could only be pushed to twenty-four per cent. Seventy-six per cent of Haitian AIDS cases remained unexplained. If we are not prepared to believe this data, which of course supports all the other data relating to Haitian AIDS patients, what price truth in AIDS research?

Heroin users

Maria threw her plaited black hair back over her shoulder and leaned forward to light another cigarette. She was casually but smartly dressed and still an attractive woman despite eighteen years as an intravenous drug user and a two-year diagnosis of AIDS. 'Does he want to talk to you about your fast-track lifestyle, mommy?' asked her son, who is seven years old.

Maria, a Puerto Rican, grew up in Harlem in an area where drug use is a commonplace occurrence, street drug dealers as common as grocery stores. No special shame was attached to drug use – families who did not have drug users in the appartment would be particularly proud of it but families with drug users would accept it as the norm, much as working class families in Europe accept heavy drinking.

Maria is in the middle of three generations of drug users; her mother is an addict and sells 'crack' to Maria's fifteen-year-old daughter, who is pregnant. One assumes scenes of unspeakable squalor and in truth Harlem is not the most refined area of Manhattan. But there is still a pride in self and the achievements of children even among junkies and prostitutes. People have to be very low before the spirit dies and in Harlem they are still fighting.

Even AIDS can be assimilated. The neighbours in Maria's building were avoiding her, knowing she had AIDS.

> I realised that everybody in the building was talking about it because I felt funny when I came out of the building, they'd be standing there and they'd look and start whispering.
>
> So one day I was upstairs and I looked out of the window and all of the mothers were standing on the stoop. I said to myself this is when I'm gonna approach these ladies and I'm gonna tell them what this is about because I had a feeling that if I didn't there was gonna be bad repercussions behind it.

So I went downstairs and I spoke to all of them and they asked me questions. They asked me about my kids and were they all right and about exactly how the virus is, is it contagious, stuff like that. I told them everything and I haven't gotten any bad response, there's no hostility.

As has been mentioned, US drug addicts were probably the first group to develop AIDS but their high mortality rate, tendency to poverty and lack of health care meant the illness was not picked up in them. Heroin itself depresses the cough response and thus makes users more likely to die of pneumonia and other chest infections – they can't cough out the phlegm. An exotic pneumonia caused by Pneumocystis carinii would not be distinguishable in a dead addict from any other kind of pneumonia which had caused death while drugs were being used. It would be just another junkie overdose.

Additionally, it is one of the peculiarities of the epidemic that surface Kaposi's sarcoma lesions are almost never seen in drug addicts, so that visual clues would not be apparent.

Addicts are also quite used to being ill with itches, rashes and a series of blood-borne diseases. The way Maria found out she had AIDS was the way many female addicts did – she had a baby and it was sick.

When my little baby was born, the first five months she got sick three times where she got high fevers and she wasn't responding to the antibiotics.

I had her in the hospital where I'd been admitted so many times, they'd saved my life there three or four times because of the infections I had got through IV drug abuse so they knew I was a drug abuser.

They approached me and told me there was a possibility that the baby could have the virus and if she got it she must have got it from me because her father is not a drug abuser.

The baby had a form of paediatric AIDS but her semi-developed immune system was fighting back and by fifteen months she had recovered. The differences between adult and child immune systems mean children, particularly young children, frequently throw off infections which would kill adults. The cancers of childhood are particularly amenable to treatment where the cancers of adulthood kill.

Maria is weak, easily fatigued, a prey to opportunistic infections but had not yet suffered Pneumocystis carinii pneumonia. Half of all women AIDS patients are IV drug users. More than seventy per cent of paediatric AIDS cases are in the children of IV drug users.

Drugs and politics

It is attractive to see drug addicts only as degenerate outcasts who have cut themselves off by their own moral failings from the succour and protection of society. This superior view was responsible for the failure of authorities to detect and deal with AIDS in drug addicts at the beginning of the epidemic. This view also fails to acknowledge the role of the Western European powers and later the US in the promotion and trade of hard drugs.

Opium use goes back as far as recorded history – Assyrian cuneiform writings refer to opium, which was known as 'lion fat', presumably a reference to its strength and to its white, fatty appearance when it is bled from incisions in the opium poppy fruit.

Morphine, a much more potent drug than raw opium, was first isolated from it by the German chemist F. W. A. Sertürner in 1806. It relieves pain and causes relaxation and calmness and is considerably less euphoric than heroin. This was first synthesised by the Englishman C. R. Wright in 1874 but his early tests on dogs showed effects which so dismayed him that he discontinued the work. The German company Bayer went further, they gave it the name Heroin from 'heroisch' which means powerful. It was marketed as a cough suppressant, a pain reliever, a universal panacea. From 1898 for more than twenty years Bayer made huge profits from their medicine until the increasing understanding of addiction led to the banning of the import and manufacture of heroin in 1924 in the US and in most of the rest of the world in succeeding years.

There were 200,000 addicts in the US at this time and the illegal purchase of drugs, or withdrawal, were the only options. The illegality of drug use led to drugs finding their place among petty criminals which of course meant among the poor.

It is estimated that at any one time a half of one per cent of the population is addicted to the strongest drug easily obtainable. Among the middle class, therefore, there is addiction to alcohol in half to one per cent in Western countries. In the UK, for example, with 56,000,000 people, there are about half a million alcoholics. In societies where heroin is the strongest drug easily obtainable – basically the ghettoes of Western countries – heroin is the principal drug of addiction. There is an association between poverty in rich countries and drug addiction, though by no means everyone who is poor and has access to the drug becomes an addict. Other factors, perhaps the much-postulated 'addictive personality', must play a part. Certainly there are also people who, however rich they are, will seek out the most powerful drug and become addicted to it in a process which seems to their families to have the inevitability of a Greek tragedy.

Empires have risen and fallen amid clouds of opium smoke. The British Empire in particular owed a great deal to drug addiction. In the eighteenth and early nineteenth centuries the British Empire was not so much a list of national possessions overseas as a flotilla of traders backed by the British navy. 'British interests abroad' were British trading interests; 'protecting British interests' meant using military power to ensure favourable trading rights.

The British East India Company was the greatest of the armed trading bodies. It required immense sums to maintain its hold over a country as vast as India and to finance its purchases of luxury goods like silk and tea which could be sent on to England. China was wealthy and almost uncharted as far as trading was concerned.

The Company established a monopoly of opium cultivation in Bengal and developed methods of cultivation of opium – applying the most advanced agricultural techniques which had been developed in the growing of less heady crops. The opium thus produced at an economical rate was sold to China for gold and silver which were used to purchase Chinese goods. In 1838 40,000 chests of opium were imported into China where the cultivation of opium was outlawed. Levels of opium addiction in China became so high that the Ch'ing dynasty itself was threatened. The Chinese government confiscated all opium warehoused at Canton by British merchants and the British sent in the fleet – the first Opium War (1838–42). This did not legalise the opium trade in China but halted Chinese attempts to stop it. The second Opium War of 1856–60 compelled China to accept the trade which escalated and weakened the Ch'ing dynasty until its fall in 1911.

The involvement of the American Empire in opium is scarcely more uplifting. Out of gratitude to the Mafia for assisting the allied effort in Sicily, the US government had Mafia boss 'Lucky' Luciano released from jail and returned to Italy in 1946. He promptly started supplying the US underworld with heroin which was first diverted from the Italian pharmaceutical industry then imported directly from Asia in the form of morphine base which Luciano's laboratories would refine into heroin for export to the US.

In Marseilles, France, in 1947, 80,000 workers came out on strike to protest about a drop in living standards. The US Central Intelligence Agency (CIA) was concerned about the growth of communism in Europe. It supplied money and arms to the Guerini brothers, Corsican gangland leaders, who attacked picket lines and union officials until the strike collapsed. In 1950 the same thing happened over a strike of Marseilles dock workers who had decided to boycott freighters supplying the French Indochinese War zone – already a developing area of US interest. The political power the Guerinis developed from this siding with the establishment and doing their dirty work allowed them to set up an immense apparatus for importing morphine and manufacturing heroin. They supplied Lucky Luciano who imported the product into the US via the Mafia network – this was the so-called 'French connection' which was supplying drugs to America throughout the fifties, sixties and early seventies. By the seventies, however, the 'French connection' was falling apart because of the decline in fortune of the Guerinis, the rise of their rivals, pressure from the US on Turkey to reduce opium production and competition from other clients of the good old CIA.

By 1970 the US was deeply and miserably involved in the Vietnam War which had such devastating social and political consequences for America and didn't do much for Vietnam, either. The object of fighting a war in Indochina was predicated on what was called the 'domino theory'. This said that once one country in an area went communist, the others would follow like one standing domino toppling into another. This was always said to be total nonsense by those opposed to the war – a racist assumption that all countries full of yellow people are alike and can be treated in exactly the same way regardless of local circumstances. It did, however, mean that more than a little attention was paid to the neighbours of Vietnam: Thailand, Cambodia, Laos.

The 'Golden Triangle' of parts of Burma, Thailand and Laos comprises the richest opium-producing region in the world. Almost all the illegal opium on the world market comes from here – 1185 tons a year in the early nineteen-seventies as compared to one hundred tons from Turkey. The Golden Triangle is very close to the border of North Vietnam.

It was essential to the American war effort to keep Laos as friendly as possible. In particular the hill tribes who were growing the opium and the armed traders who were acting as intermediaries between the producers and the Dutch smugglers of the drug had to be placated. If their livelihood were threatened, they would be easy prey to communist influences. They were, however, at present not well disposed towards North Vietnam whose puritanical opposition to opium was well known. The CIA therefore protected the opium growers and shippers from the influence of the Indochinese governments at the same time as the Federal Bureau of Narcotics was putting pressure on these governments to control the cultivation of opium. They armed the traders and gave free passage to the smugglers. I do not believe that the CIA actually transported the drugs themselves as is sometimes claimed.

The opium thus produced was refined into morphine blocks near the fields, then smuggled in this form (it is bulkier but more difficult for dogs to detect than heroin) into Amsterdam or Paris then into the USA where it would go into the veins of young Americans. Other blocks would go to Hong Kong to be refined and then would be smuggled back to Indochina, to Saigon, where it would find its way into the hands of dealers supplying American servicemen and then into the veins of other young Americans.

The high percentage of drug addicts among American soldiers significantly contributed to the drug problem in the US and indirectly, therefore, to the spread of AIDS.

Heroin use and AIDS

The number of intravenous drug users with AIDS has stabilised in the US and in the twenty-eight countries of the World Health Organization's AIDS survey at around twenty per cent of the total. If AIDS were going to burst out of the main risk categories, it would be expected that the percentage covered by this rather small drug subculture would decline progressively as AIDS in the non-risk groups increased – this has yet to occur. A leading article in the *British Medical Journal* in February 1987 was titled 'AIDS and intravenous drug use: the real heterosexual epidemic.'

Some researchers have implicated drugs, because of their role in suppressing the immune system, in AIDS cases in addition to those where the patient is a declared IV drug user. Cesar Caceres, now a Washington doctor but formerly with the US Public Health Service, noted that, 'since the CDC lists intravenous drug users below homosexual and bisexual men, it classified AIDS patients as IV drug users only if they are exclusively IV drug users. If we add the homosexual and bisexual IV drug users to the exclusively heterosexual drug users we find at least twenty-five per cent of AIDS patients have been intravenous drug users.'

When he adds in patients who have taken recreational drugs orally, culled from CDC studies of patients, it is apparent that seventy-nine per cent of AIDS patients have been drug users.

'Since drug abuse can severely damage the immune system, why has AIDS been identified primarily with sex, especially sex among homosexuals?'

This is, of course, going too far. The amount to which marijuana damages the immune system, if at all, is widely open to question. One cannot, either, compare the occasional or even frequent use of 'soft' recreational drugs with the permanently drugged state of the heroin addict.

There are, however, a couple of highly significant points in Caceres' analysis: hard drugs do damage the immune system, rendering it more open to infection by any agent and 'most people who have contracted AIDS, whatever their sexual orientation, have led a "fast-track" lifestyle involving sexual experimentation, promiscuity and drug abuse.'

Darrell Yates Rist, who knows a great deal about Greenwich Village street life, comments that some gays who frequented bars and bath houses would get an occasional 'high' from heroin just as a special treat. 'These guys would need needles but they couldn't just go in and buy them at a store, so an underground business grew up in selling them. They were sold and packaged as new because these guys wanted clean needles for the reasons of ordinary hygiene but in fact they were old needles that were just washed and packaged to look like new. They could have been carrying anything.'

This was an unknowing sharing of needles and of any pathogens the last user had. A more unsettling practice, at least for those outside the drug world, is the practice of sharing needles. In the so-called 'shooting galleries' up to sixty people could be injected with the same needle before it became too blunt for use. The most anonymous contact with this inoculum would be when someone spoke to a look-out and tout standing outside, say, an abandoned building. The would-be high would walk in to the building and stick his arm through a hole in the wall. Someone on the other side would take the money from the hand and inject it but neither would see the other so the risk of betrayal to narcotics agents would be minimal.

Slightly more convivial but probably still in an abandoned building would be the gathering where a number of addicts would hand over money – say $10 each – and the friendly local dealer with his own 'works' would inject one person after another. An advantage of doing this for addicts with collapsed veins in all accessible parts of their body would be that someone else could inject them in areas they couldn't reach themselves. There was, I am told, an additional fee for this service.

Much more frequent would be the friendly gathering of people who knew each other well and who bought, sold or loaned drugs amongst themselves and who regularly shared needles, because of their short supply.

Recognising that some people will share needles, whatever the advice, organisations like the Mid City Consortium to Combat AIDS in San Francisco attempt to work within the addicts' own culture. George Williams was an addict for fourteen years. Now he works for the Mid City Consortium along with other ex-addicts and ex-prostitutes to attempt to control the growth of AIDS. San Francisco, as one of the more enduring aspects of the summer of love, has an extremely high rate of drug use – there are 12,000 intravenous drug users in the city. George's patch is the notorious Tenderloin district where the street people, almost exclusively black, hang around in the afternoon sun, just rapping or waiting for the man.

For some reason work with drug addicts in Europe is concentrated in the hands of social workers and doctors. The US has a vigorous tradition of employing people who really know the scene.

George said:

We're all ex-hypes or ex-hookers. I got off junk because it was just time for me to, I was in detox and I had been cleaned up many times before but this time I decided to stay straight.

These here are my people and I love them. They welcome me because they know I'm not laying any shit on them – I'm just helping them to avoid AIDS. I give them each a bottle of bleach to clean the syringe with, and rubbers so they don't pass AIDS on if they got it or get it from anyone else.

Street workers like George have encouraged addicts to build the use of bleach into the ritual of drug use – they fill the syringe and empty it twice between different users. It should kill off any pathogen and is at least an effective method of prevention where simply telling people not to use intravenous drugs is not.

The reason for this sharing of drug tools is that possession of the 'works' is itself a crime in eleven states and the District of Columbia. While this may not seem a great many from fifty states and DC, the states are all those which have high drug use and, inevitably, are those which have a high level of AIDS, including the AIDS centres of New York, New Jersey, California and Illinois.

People with the public good at heart, but little knowledge of human behaviour, enacted these laws in the belief that fewer needles would mean less drug addiction. Instead, sharing became commonplace – indeed, rituals developed around sharing – and a considerable problem had been created with hepatitis being transmitted in this fashion long before AIDS.

Vince Morrone who is researching the subject for the Committee on Health of the New York State Assembly said: 'I defy anyone to find a public health official worth his salt who feels that making the possession of needles a criminal act reduces the rate of addiction.

'These laws remain because they carry weight with the political people. If the District Attorney said he wanted to see needles become available to drug abusers, that would be political death.'

Europe and drug use

The European approach is somewhat different. In most Western European countries, if not all of them, needles and syringes are easily available. If there had been reservations about selling needles to addicts in the past, pharmacists have no such qualms now. In some areas a needle exchange scheme is operating – in Amsterdam a needle brought in to a methadone clinic by an addict will be replaced with a new one. Methadone is a kind of synthetic heroin designed to replace heroin in addicts' lives. In fact it has become just another drug for sale and distribution on the streets, so in some areas, like Holland, where it is available it must be taken at the clinic. The system in Amsterdam is now used by thirty to fifty per cent of opiate injectors and has not increased the incidence of needle use. Similar needle-exchange pilot schemes have been set up in a number of British cities, notably Edinburgh where an apparent shortage of needles early in the AIDS epidemic period led to a great deal of sharing.

Britain, with 50,000 daily heroin users and about the same number of casual users, has seized on the AIDS epidemic to reinforce an anti-heroin message directed at the young who have been increasingly using heroin, first in the crude 'brown sugar' form which can be smoked, then in the more purified (though never more than ten per cent pure) forms which are injected. Anti-drug ads concentrated on the deception and petty theft of addicts, often directed against members of their own family. Personal degradation – a girl vomiting in a lavatory bowl or being paid for sexual services in a dingy room – was also thought to be a particular turn-off for the young. The government campaign was attempting to discourage the first use of a syringe – which would almost inevitably be with someone else's works – and to discourage sex with addicts. 'If a smack-head tries to chat you up, what's he really after?' cleverly tried to discourage girls from having sexual contact with addicts by implying that a drug addict did not want sex but in fact was really interested in 'what he can scrounge or nick off you'.

Inevitably some self-righteous conservatives had to attack the campaign. Member of Parliament Teddy Taylor took particular exception to the disarming: 'It only takes one prick to give you AIDS.'

He said: 'A lot of people have been worried about the publicity used in this campaign. Most advertisers will agree that it is perfectly possible to shock people without causing unnecessary offence. This particular advertisement, like some of its predecessors, seems to go over the top. I do not see how it is going to help potential sufferers from AIDS.'

It is unfortunate that some people would not recognize the central importance of addicts, sex with addicts and needles. Drug addicts are the bridging group which crosses all the other groups and goes out into the free country of the uninfected like a highway.

It is possible that drug addicts had AIDS first and then passed it into the homosexual community. This cannot be known for certain but most definitely the overlap between homosexuals and drug addicts over the use of needles in order to enjoy this devastating drug recreationally will have increased the level of AIDS infection in the homosexual community. Homosexual prostitution among drug addicts is another area of overlap but they would be most likely to be the 'passive' partners and thus at more risk of infection than of infecting others.

Infected addicts would pass AIDS on to heterosexual partners. Women addicts would infect their children and perhaps, if prostitutes, the 'Johns', though this is a most unlikely route of infection as will be discussed.

Haitian American immigrants would be in the same social circumstances as the majority of drug addicts: poor, living in slums, sometimes involved in crime. Their connection with the drug addicts would be more tenuous but there would have been some overlap.

Much more important is the connection with haemophiliacs via plasmapheresis centres where drug addicts would be paid to pass on their infected plasma which would be used and would contaminate whole batches of Factor VIII, which would then be sold on the open market around the world, infecting Europe, Japan, you name it.

Both in terms of their own disease and in terms of its spread, drug addicts have suffered in all countries from their lack of organisation and lack of leadership. Long after it was realised there was a serious problem, nothing was done for addicts. Advice to prevent the spread of AIDS has been slow to arrive and limited in its outlook. Very little advice has been given to addicts about, for example, the necessity of using condoms. This is presumably because of a one-dimensional picture of addicts in which they are presented as dope fiends with no contact with everyday life except through the barrel of a syringe. The fact that drug addicts have families, lovers and are often employed in marginal jobs did not seem to penetrate the minds of the agencies, generally government agencies, which were finally called to respond to the needs of this despised 'problem group'.

Les Papas, himself a former addict, works for the San Fransisco AIDS Foundation making contact with intravenous drug users. He said: 'I think people have a perception of drug addicts as being very fatalistic, self-destructive, people who don't care about themselves or anyone else. What we've found is that, the more we work with them, we realise those are not accurate perceptions. Drug addicts are real people, just like anyone else. They care about themselves and they care about other people in their lives. We've seen that concern and we've been able to measure the changes that they've made in not sharing needles and cleaning needles and using condoms. I think that suggests they don't want to die, they don't want to be sick, they don't want to give AIDS to anyone else. They're human and need to be treated as such, they have a desire to live, they're not all out to kill themselves.'

Resources were available to haemophiliacs through existing organisations; Haitians at least had a government batting for them; homosexuals were already organised and finally persuaded governments to take action and even to fund their projects to help AIDS patients. Drug addicts have and have had no speakers and few supporters. They have even found themselves vilified by other organisations for AIDS victims. Gay Men's Health Crisis will not work with drug addicts who are not in a detoxification programme. They enraged Joe Sonnabend by ordering one of their volunteer 'buddies' to stop working with a junkie.

Joe Sonnabend is as eager as any doctor to get junkies off dope or at least on to methadone but it is hard to find structured programmes for every addict who needs them, particularly when the addict is ill and cannot travel far. It is most unlikely that addicts will go through withdrawal when they have AIDS and are in particular need of the solace of drugs. The presentation of withdrawal as an unimaginable horror is a junkie myth – though it's not fun, it's not that bad – but even a mildly unpleasant experience would not be something an addict with AIDS would want to walk into. Sonnabend kept prescribing drugs, the Gay Men's Health Crisis told the buddy to stop visiting the addict, the buddy refused but instead stopped visiting Gay Men's Health Crisis.

A sensible and compassionate approach to drug addiction early enough in the epidemic would have considerably reduced the risk of the further spread of AIDS.

Homosexuals

Gay Monopoly advertises itself as 'A celebration of gay life' and it offers everything the makers want to feel good about: the board is decorated with drawings of leather-clad young men with moustaches, players use small models of a leather cap, a hair dryer, manacles. The 'properties' they can buy are homosexual haunts like Spruce Street, Philadelphia, or Clark Street, Chicago. They are challenged with cards requiring them to guess the name from a brief biography of great homosexuals of yesteryear, such as Hans Christian Andersen and John Maynard Keynes. The other 'quiz' cards expect a player to guess the meaning of a coloured hanky when worn dangling from the pocket of a tight pair of jeans: light blue in the left pocket means the wearer wants fellatio, in the right pocket means the wearer wants to give oral sex; pink in the left pocket means the wearer likes to use dildos, in the right it means he likes to have them used on him. Players can collect bars on the 'properties' and if they have four bars they can buy a bathhouse. Proceeds from the sale of *Gay Monopoly* go to AIDS charities.

Homosexuality is as old as mankind and has frequently been accepted even more freely than it has in Western countries in recent years. Attitudes towards homosexuality appear to have followed Matthew Arnold's division of Western civilisation by its two great influences: the Hellenic and the Hebraic. Greek civilisation and the Persians and Romans who were influenced by it tolerated and even praised homosexuality. Jewish and later Christian cultures abominated homosexuality though it was always present as an undercurrent even from the Middle Ages to the end of the nineteenth century when the Church was strong in Europe. Homosexuals wishing to establish their tradition have always been keen to refer back to Plato, citing liberal scholars like E. M. Forster and Oscar Wilde as they go back through the centuries, seeking authorities to justify their sexual preference.

Homosexuals are a large minority. Alfred Kinsey in 1948 estimated that there were four per cent of American males who were exclusively homosexual, ten per cent who were for at least three years of their lives and thirty per cent who had had an adult homosexual experience leading to orgasm. It is generally accepted that there are at least ten million male homosexuals in the USA.

An increasing atmosphere of freedom in the nineteen-sixties led to the rise of liberation movements for many minority groups (and for women – a majority group) with homosexual men and women in the forefront of protests against police repression and to subsequent 'gay pride' consciousness. The 'Gay Liberation' movement is dated from Friday 27 June 1969 at the Stonewall Inn on New York's Christopher Street. This was an area where many homosexuals congregated and because of this the New York police delighted in turning up to harass them, particularly the transvestites. The difference on this warm summer night was that when New York's finest arrived to raid the Stonewall Inn for alleged infringement of liquor laws, the gay patrons fought back. Police reinforcements were sent in and it was time for a show-down. Rioting continued over three days and while it is probably true to say that the police 'won', gay pride had asserted itself; homosexual areas were left to flourish.

Between the late nineteen-sixties and the early nineteen-seventies most liberal nations removed legal restraints on homosexual acts (*being* a homosexual had never been an offence, only specific practices) though the authoritarian Catholic and Communist countries retained prohibitions. Most states also maintained a different age of consent for heterosexuals – generally the age of consent for homosexual acts had been twenty-one, while the age of consent for heterosexual acts had been sixteen. In some cases anomalies were left – when homosexual acts were legalised in Great Britain in 1967, the old law forbidding sodomy remained, so it is still 'a felony for a person to commit buggery with another person' even if the other person is his wife. The law as it related to men was superseded but not as it related to women. There have been no recent prosecutions.

There had been civil rights movements before gay liberation, aimed at lifting the legal restraints to homosexual acts and, as we have seen, they were largely successful. Had this been all, and the homosexual world had settled down into a series of monogamous relationships culminating in man and husband living happily ever after, AIDS would not have spread with any speed in the homosexual community. Gay liberation was the missing psychological factor which turned homosexuals from people at slightly elevated risk for AIDS into super vectors whose society would be laid waste by it.

The fundamental difference between gay liberation and its civil rights predecessors, Dennis Altman maintains in his book *Homosexual Oppression and Liberation*, was that the civil rights movements wanted homosexuals to be accepted, they were as good as straight society, they should not be discriminated against on the grounds of what they did with their genitals.

For the gay power movement, 'no longer is the claim made that gay people can fit into American society, that they are as decent, as patriotic, as clean living as anyone else. Rather, it is argued, it is American Society itself that needs to change.' This was a running theme of the liberation movements of the late sixties and early seventies. Black people did not need more rights, they needed the whole of white society to stop being racist and preventing them from developing their own culture; women demanded society be less sexist; the schoolkids movement and the 'Grey Panthers' for older people wanted society to be less ageist; pacifists demanded it be less militarist.

Homosexuals wanted a redefinition of what was acceptable sexual behaviour. Homosexuality was not to be seen as a deviation but as a normal state of being, albeit for a minority of the population. Once there was the freedom to be openly homosexual, at least in some areas like New York's Christopher Street and San Francisco's Castro Street, what was to be done with this freedom? This approaches the question of what is a homosexual? Presumably someone who performs or wants to perform homosexual acts. To have one's life defined by sexuality is much more rare in heterosexual society and it could be argued that it never occurs, that the pin-up and prostitute and male stripper and model are just doing a job and 'are' someone independent of their sexual status. Homosexuals are what they do with their bodies. And they did.

Bathhouses had existed in a furtive form in most big cities before gay lib. Then they 'came out'. Dennis Altman describes them:

> These resemble nothing so much as giant steaming whorehouses in which everyone is a customer; clad only in white towels men prowl the hallways, groping each other in furtive search for instant sex, making it in small, dark cubicles on low, hard, come-stained beds. Disgusting? – yes, perhaps. Yet lasting friendships are quite commonly begun in bathhouses and to this extent the whorehouse analogy is not fully accurate. It is a feature of male homosexual life that sex usually precedes intimacy to a much greater extent than among heterosexuals.

Altman is being characteristically coy about treading on anyone's sexual feelings. In fact sex preceding intimacy would occur with far greater frequency in heterosexual relationships were it not for the sexual reserve of women, a restraint homosexual men were relieved of.

Whether because of upbringing or innate distaste is immaterial, it is demonstrable that men find the idea of repeated acts of anonymous sex exciting and women do not. Women given the opportunity to have sex with a number of men in a short space of time tend not to do it. Men in the same position do. The promiscuity of the homosexual scene in the nineteen-seventies was a product of male sexuality given free licence, not of homosexuality exclusively.

Even at the height of liberation in the nineteen-seventies women were hardly involved at all in the sort of behaviour described in *Faggots*, a novel published in 1978 by Larry Kramer, later to become famous for founding the Gay Men's Health Crisis in response to AIDS and writing the play *The Normal Heart* about the early months of the epidemic.

Faggots tells the story of Fred Lemish, a film scriptwriter, in his quest for love amid the bars, bathhouses and beaches of homosexual New York. In that it is about love amid scenarios of sex, it achieves the tricky task of being both a sentimental and a pornographic novel. Other characters include Randy Dildough, the sadistic executive; Winnie Heinz, the ageing male model; Timmy Purvis, the beautiful young boy from out West and Abe Bronstein, the movie financier whom Fred is attempting to persuade to back a romantic film about homosexuals.

Early in the novel Kramer offers a client's-eye-view of the bathhouse scene:

Fred stood there helplessly. Why was he inert in a moment requiring action? The guy wasn't bad-looking. Should Fred enter, or walk away?

'Fuck my friend and I'll suck your come out of his asshole.'

This suggestion Fred recognised as 'felching'. Was he interested in joining a felcher?

'Or I could tie you up. Or you could tie us up. Or either one of us. Or anything else your cock desires!'

The man certainly offered a range of choices. Should Fred? Shouldn't Fred?

'Are you into shit?'

Fred shouldn't.

Why was he even hesitating, Fred asked himself, instead of just walking on? Because he was horny, that's why, and this guy looked better than anybody else, there not being many here this afternoon anyway, and he wanted to get it over with and leave.

Fred does, of course. In another encounter that day Fred, who is not presented in the book as being particularly promiscuous, compared to other characters, has sex with a man in a public lavatory during which a third man breaks open a 'popper' and offers it to Fred's nostrils at the point of orgasm.

Observers of the homosexual scene have commented not only on the frequency of sexual encounters but on their anonymity. As one *Faggots* character comments to another, with heterosexual encounters, even with a prostitute, a few words are exchanged: 'Hallo, what's your name, where are you from, how much do you charge?' Even these pleasantries are lacking in homosexual encounters on the streets or in the bars. A 'safe sex' publication from San Francisco, *The Hot 'n' Healthy Times*, suggests repartee for post-AIDS contacts:

'"I'd love to play with your ass," says the hot hunk you've just met over a beer.

'"That would be great!" you immediately respond. Then after an awkward pause: "But we've got to use condoms."'

This suggests that when boy meets boy in San Francisco, at least in the new era, a few words are exchanged, even if they are a little lacking in lyricism.

When AIDS hit the homosexual communities of the US, several studies were conducted by the vigilant CDC to determine what it was in the homosexual lifestyle which predisposed to this immunosuppressive condition. There were really only two things which distinguished the homosexual lifestyle: the promiscuous sex and the extensive use of recreational drugs.

Looking at homosexual men with and without the disease it looked clear that the AIDS patients were mainly those who had a large number of sexual contacts (and 'large' often meant twenty a week); those who were receptive to anal intercourse and those who practised 'fist fucking' or 'brachioproctal intercourse'. This was a trend and not universally true – nothing ever is in medicine and epidemiology. Some people with few sexual partners had AIDS, some with many sexual partners did not, some men who were 'active' in anal intercourse also contracted AIDS. While the early researchers were surprised at the number of sexual partners the sick (and healthy) men had, sex had been around for a long time and hadn't caused these sorts of problems before. On the other hand, sex at the level at which these men enjoyed it, involving so many people, was new. For just over a decade it was possible for anyone, waiters and diplomats and building workers, to enjoy orgies every night at a level which had previously been known to a very few individuals throughout human history – the Roman Emperor Tiberius's antics at Capri suggest themselves, or the erotic pleasures of Emperor Yang Ti of the Sui Dynasty in China. Moreover, even the great debauchees of the past had not been so frequently receptive of semen as the New York gays were. In general they had been rampant males being satisfied with a series of females, not anally receptive males or females. The only historical example I can think of where a person has become famous for being a repository of semen was Messalina, the Emperor Claudius's wife, who challenged the leading prostitute in Rome to a contest, to see who could have the most men. Messalina won.

There must have been many women who received multiple doses of semen from various men but presumably almost always vaginally. Moreover women were not developing AIDS, even those from the heterosexual swingers clubs which mirrored the bathhouses – though there were far fewer of them. Semen itself could not be a poison – people had been drinking it and women had been accepting it vaginally for too long; someone would have noticed.

Could it be the anal route? Certainly the membrane lining the rectum is far more delicate than the lining of the vagina and some promiscuous homosexuals had a tendency to sado-masochism which somewhat increased the vigour of the intercourse they engaged in – when they were engaged in intercourse rather than inserting other objects into the orifice of their choice. Up to half the AIDS patients in the first studies had been 'fisted'.

A theory grew up that there was a substance in semen which is immunosuppressive. It was identified as the enzyme transglutaminase by Richard Ablin, working with Hungarian colleagues at the State University of New York. This has been mentioned in reference to haemophiliacs who injected the enzyme in the protein which came with their Factor VIII. Homosexuals would inject it too – into the rectum and through the tears in the rectal mucosa into the bloodstream – with what has been called 'the great inoculum': the penis. This theory of the cause of AIDS has fallen from favour, the first blow being the realisation that AIDS was caused by an infectious agent – otherwise how are the cases among drug addicts and transfusion recipients explained? These had no contact with semen or transglutaminase. The second blow came when the decision was made to declare HIV and no additional thing the cause. Work on other theories and even proven facts like the undoubted immunosuppressant effects of semen when injected into the bloodstream, simply stopped.

The other theory of the cause was the drugs homosexual men used. They used rather a lot. Larry Kramer lists them in *Faggots*. Omitting his comments and the sixteen varieties of marijuana, they are: MDA, MDM, THC, PCP, STP, DMT, LDK, WDW, Coke, Window Pane, Blotter, Orange Sunshine, Sweet Pea, Sky Blue, Christmas Tree, Mescalin, Dust, Benzedrine, Dexedrine, Dexamyl, Desoxyn, Strychnine, Ionamin, Ritalin, Desbutal, Opitol, Glue, Ethyl Chloride, Nitrous Oxide, Crystal Methedrine, Clogidal, Nesperan, Tytch, Nestex, Black Beauty, Certyn, Preludin with B-12, Zayl, Quaalude, Tuinal, Nembutal, Seconal, Amytal, Phenobarb, Elavil, Valium, Librium, Darvon, Mandrax, Opium, Stidyl, Halidax, Calcifyn, Optimil, Drayl.

Once they understood the range of drug use, life was easier for the early researchers. While most men who went to the homosexual discos and bathhouses used some drugs, there were few which were commonly used. Only amyl nitrite and butyl nitrite were used by a large number of AIDS patients – more than ninety per cent. These are drugs sold in the form of small phials which can be opened and sniffed or smaller containers which can be smashed and sniffed – good for one use only.

Amyl nitrite was developed for use in people with heart disease when the pain of angina occurs. The pain is caused by a lack of oxygenated blood reaching the heart muscle. Amyl nitrite, a 'vasodilator', enlarges the blood vessels to the heart and allows more blood to reach it. It also dilates the blood vessels to the brain, causing dizziness, and to other parts of the body. In relaxing the anal sphincter, poppers made anal sex less painful and more enjoyable, also easing the passage of other objects, such as hands, into the anus.

In the investigation of the nitrites several things became clear very quickly; only butyl nitrite was freely available; it had superseded its more refined sibling when amyl went on prescription. The epidemiology of popper sniffing equals AIDS was obviously faulty – too many people who used poppers did not have AIDS. There was also a problem of how to dissociate popper use from other aspects of homosexual lifestyle which predisposed to popper use. People who had many sexual partners, and who were anally receptive and more likely to be fisted, also used poppers. Was it one of these traits which caused AIDS or a combination of them or none of them?

The chemicals themselves were not as helpful as might have been hoped in yielding answers. Popper use suppressed the immune system in some volunteers in experiments, not in others, and in some animal experiments, though not all of them.

Animal experiments have not been helpful in AIDS research; the absence of an animal model for the whole disease makes forays into the animal kingdom with single aspects of AIDS unhelpful to the point of being misleading.

The discovery of new AIDS patients with no hint of popper use killed the popper theory, though some people find it valuable in describing the prior immune suppression of AIDS patients and the aspects of AIDS which are almost exclusive to homosexuals, like external Kaposi's sarcoma. CDC researchers dropped the poppers theory, then, because it did not fit the facts. The discipline of their behaviour at this early stage in the epidemic is impressive considering subsequent developments in AIDS research. The field workers of CDC dropped the theory because it did not fit the facts; they did not massage the facts to make them fit the theory.

So what was it about homosexuals which made them peculiarly susceptible to AIDS? Their numbers (including homosexuals or bisexuals who were also intravenous drug users) stabilised at seventy per cent of cases in the US and remained at that level. In Europe the figures were often higher: eighty-six per cent in Denmark; eighty-eight per cent in Holland; eighty-seven per cent in the UK – figures for the end of 1987. These figures are for countries with a number of AIDS cases who weren't flown in from abroad, like those in France and Belgium, where national figures became distorted. Iceland and Poland's homosexual AIDS cases are one hundred per cent of the total but the numbers of people involved are four and two respectively.

Why so many homosexuals? Peter Duesberg's advice is to 'work with the patient, go back to the clinic or back onto the streets or in the bathhouses to study those who are at risk, the haemophiliacs or the promiscuous male homosexuals or the intravenous drug users. We have to see what AIDS is, AIDS is not a disease entity, AIDS is a whole bag of old diseases under a new name.'

The champion of the theory that AIDS is 'multi-factorial' or caused by many interacting factors is Joe Sonnabend. He was born in Africa and understood the diseases which were being presented to him in his New York practice. Gut problems like giardiasis, amoebiasis and salmonellosis are not problems of people in rich, hygienic countries. He said:

> AIDS is characteristic of disease conditions in situations of deprivation and poverty when individuals are exposed to multitudes of micro-organisms, the spread of which is facilitated by crowding and poor sanitation, frequently complicated by the consequences of poor nutrition on the immune system.
>
> Among individuals in Western countries who have developed AIDS there has frequently been the creation of circumstances that approximate to the conditions in developing countries. For example in highly interactive promiscuous settings where multiple sex partners are the rule, sexual interchanges become highly contaminated with common sexually transmitted organisms. These individuals are going to be bombarded with pathogenic micro-organisms.

To put it more explicitly: an even better way to get gut parasites than drinking infected water is to lick someone's anus or suck someone's penis after it has been up another person's rectum. Having repeated sexual partners passing round the same micro-organisms means repeated reinfection by, for example, cytomegalovirus, each time in a slightly different form as the virus itself evolves. When fifty of the early AIDS patients were tested for antibodies to various infections, all of them had cytomegalo and Epstein-Barr viruses, which are known to be immunosuppressive. All had herpes simplex I and forty-nine had herpes simplex II. Forty-seven had hepatitis B antibodies. The control group of other men from the same milieu had almost the same pattern of disease.

Treatments for disease could also be immunosuppressive – repeated doses of antibiotics and drugs like metronidazole which is given for bowel problems could also be related to AIDS. Or perhaps repeated reinfection when treatment was not completed meant the pathogens were strengthened – treatment killed off the weakest strains and left the strongest to flourish, leaving the immune system open to greater attack. Whatever the cause of AIDS, single or multi-factorial, it is certain that the promiscuous homosexuals of the late seventies and early eighties were fertile ground for an epidemic.

Darrell Yates Rist commented on the attitude of homosexuals to sexually transmitted diseases before AIDS:

> When a gay graduate school mate of mine couldn't shake hepatitis B in 1975, I chalked it up, with condescending pity, to bad genes. 'Some

people,' I mused glibly, 'die young of colds.' Survival of the fittest.
That year, several thousand men, women and children died of
complications due to hepatitis B. Gay men were a high-risk group.
They still are, constituting twenty-nine per cent of the cases. . . . But
unlike AIDS, hepatitis hasn't captured much of anyone's imagi-
nation. Since it was around before the liberated visibility of
homosexuals, it's never latched its hideous identity to any exotic
group enough to get its due attention. And so its victims scream, but
silently.

The homosexual community did not immediately leap into action
when it became apparent there was an epidemic of a new syndrome in
their midst. They ignored it and hoped it would go away. While a small
number of doctors and activists like Larry Kramer were ringing
warning bells and collecting money for research, throughout 1981 the
epidemic was spreading and very little attention was being paid to it.
Being gay was about youth and beauty and good health, being sick
didn't fit in.

When the connections were first made between homosexual
behaviour and AIDS, the homosexual community reacted with anger
and denial: centuries of oppression had culminated in a state of liberty
which was not going to be jeopardised by a few suspicious deaths. They
were prepared to blame anything for AIDS in order to defend the
sanctity of anal sex. The fear was that the right wing, the so-called
'moral majority' in the US, would use the nascent epidemic as an excuse
to attack homosexuals.

Slowly, safer-sex suggestions were accepted by the gay community,
then enthusiastically endorsed as more people died. The Gay Men's
Health Crisis newsletter *The Volunteer* offers evenings with films 'that
make safer sex positively erotic', workshops on 'mastering safer S/M
sex' and anecdotes which indicate all was not gloom: like the time when
an extremely explicit safer-sex workshop was, due to a misrouting of
public address system cables, broadcast to the bar mitzvah celebrations
in a nearby function room.

Darryl Yates Rist visited the Mine Shaft, one of the best-known
homosexual night spots, in the safer-sex era:

> In darkness broken only by the red glow of the exit lights, men are
> masturbating: a whack against someone's behind, a wrenching pinch
> on someone's tits, the obligatory 'yeah', an urgent groan, spasmodic
> sighs. One man's kneeling on the floor. Though he's walking on the
> health code's razor edge, he's only tonguing balls. Neither cock nor
> come are in his mouth – a distinction sex inspectors might not care to

make. Downstairs on the damp, ground floor, three of four bathtubs formerly used for watersports are covered, in compliance with the guidelines from a gay group named 'The Coalition for Sexual Responsibility'. In one tub which the management has not yet sealed a man is on his knees. There's no evidence that watersports can transmit AIDS but this man isn't taking chances. A steady stream of piss is washing on his chest but he doesn't let any near his mouth.

The 'health code' referred to is the New York State's Public Health Council resolution of 25 October 1985, forbidding anal intercourse and fellatio in 'any place in which entry, membership, goods or services are purchased'. While publicly promoted as a measure to prevent the spread of AIDS, in fact the powers conferred on health inspectors were almost exclusively used against homosexuals. Darryl Yates Rist also visited the heterosexual Plato's Retreat and found 'safer sex' wasn't an issue, 'seven women gave their partners blow jobs in plain view . . . one woman in the orgy room was getting it – two men at once, no condoms, front and back.'

Certainly there was nothing special about gay sex in terms of its capacity to pass on pathogenic organisms. What was special was the frequency of sexual encounters.

Much of the hostility directed at homosexuals is at base envy for their sexual range. When AIDS came it was attractive to the dully monogamous heterosexuals to see HIV antibody positivity as a mark of Cain – they might be well now but they would soon die. As Peter Duesberg said: 'The conservatives say look at all these guys. They've been doing all these things and they're still alive, I've been doing two dates a year, what have I been missing?' It was curiously comforting for those who had never been sexually free to think that all those who had were going to die a horrible death.

Support for concerted action against AIDS only began to grow when it was clear heterosexuals could be affected. As US Secretary of Health and Human Services Margaret Heckler said at the first International Conference on AIDS in Atlanta in April 1985: 'We must conquer (AIDS) before it infects the heterosexual population and threatens the health of the general population.' Homosexual activists interpreted this to mean if only faggots and niggers were dying that was OK but if real people started to die then something had to be done.

Randy Shilts's book *And the Band Played On* offers a moving and intimate picture of San Francisco as the plague hit the homosexual community. Shilts is angry about so many things, it is difficult to isolate the strands: lack of research funding; squabbling between scientists; lack of funding for care facilities for AIDS victims; anti-homosexual prejudice and the failure of the rest of the country to pay attention when young men were dying in their thousands. Overwhelmingly, however, and uniquely in that book, Shilts tells how gay politics were so centred on sexuality that the great issue which divided the homosexual community and turned friends into bitter enemies in San Francisco was whether the bathhouses should be closed.

Their political consciousness was so bound up with the open expression of their sexuality that the great battle was fought over plans to close the bathhouses.

For many gay activists, the bathhouse culture symbolised everything they stood for, everything they had fought for. For them, if you didn't go to the baths, you were in the closet. Those who wanted the baths closed were described as 'sexual fascists' and 'homophobes'. The arguments in their favour were that the baths were the places where the promiscuous homosexuals went and were therefore the places where AIDS education could best be put across. Visits to these establishments in 1984 convinced public health inspectors that even if education about AIDS was available at the bathhouses, the patrons were not heeding it. The bathhouses were not closed down until October 1984 in San Francisco, in the city where the first AIDS cases had been diagnosed almost four years earlier.

The homosexual community's leaders also suffered the maladies of all single-issue pressure groups: political in-fighting and an obsession with nomenclature. It became a major issue that articles about AIDS should not use 'judgmental' terms like 'promiscuous' and that people with AIDS should not be referred to as 'patients' or 'victims': 'because the semantics implied they were passive and helpless at a time when they wanted to fight actively to regain their health'. That was the petty and weak side of the homosexual reaction to the AIDS epidemic. There was also a reaction of great courage.

The *New York Native*

When Christopher Street was gay, really gay, not the sad shadowy place it is now, Chuck Ortleb looked at it and asked what it needed. He was a bright lad, a poet and activist, when he arrived in 1973 fresh from an English degree at the University of Kansas. 'I was concerned about the low level of material that was being published by and for gay people. I was part of an organisation that started a magazine called *Out* in 1973. This folded after two issues but I'd got the bug to publish and I was determined to start something else and two years later I started *Christopher Street*. This is a literary magazine.'

In the romantic, light-hearted atmosphere of Greenwich Village in the nineteen-seventies *Christopher Street* flourished. By the beginning of the eighties life was not so good for the magazine. '*Christopher Street* was going bankrupt and I thought maybe I could start another business to save it, and it worked, I started *New York Native*.'

This is a characteristic Ortleb trait: when in difficulties, open up a second front. The *Native* was a serious news and features magazine which quickly attracted some of the best gay writing talent. It was started, quite by chance, right at the beginning of the AIDS epidemic. 'We got stuck with it as our main story.'

First he hired strictly medical writers – an MD, then a PhD in microbiology, then Ann Guidici Fettner, writer of *The Truth About AIDS*. They all served the magazine well. *Native* was the only lay publication (in fact one of very few publications of any kind) which followed the AIDS story in the scientific detail it merited. 'We noticed peculiarities about that story,' said Ortleb, 'and I began to wonder whether it was a medical story or a crime story.'

Ortleb had taken the trouble to understand the science himself and he came to realise how this story could be understood in mere human terms when stripped of its jargon. *New York Native* covered earlier than any other publication the story of the competition between the French and the Americans for priority over HIV; they called it Gallogate. It covered the mysterious outbreak of AIDS in Belle Glade, Florida, which at one time in 1985 had a rate of AIDS cases more than five times that of New York City. It covered the African swine fever story with relentless thoroughness. It was in the forefront of investigation of the alleged connection between syphilis and AIDS.

New York Native was the flagship of the homosexual reaction to the AIDS epidemic. It was here that Larry Kramer, mad with indignation at the inaction of the gay community, wrote his stirring '1,112 and Counting', referring to the number of AIDS deaths.

'If this article doesn't scare the shit out of you we're in real trouble. If this article doesn't rouse you to anger, fury, rage and action, gay men may have no future on this earth. Our continued existence depends on just how angry you can get.' Doctors, epidemiologists, politicians, journalists, the patients themselves. No one was spared the lash.

Ortleb's was journalism not of the old school but of the old century. The outrage, the refusal even to consider any question of balance is reminiscent of the writing of Defoe and Swift and the great pamphleteers. Comparing the *Native* to other journals reporting the AIDS situation is like comparing a waterfall to a stagnant pond. Week after week the *Native* thundered a message of dissent, a rallying cry for all who were suspicious of the AIDS establishment.

The down side was that people who find everything suspicious and look for sinister motives in all actions of the establishment run the risk of not being taken seriously on any issue. The African swine fever story was being presented as a great scandal and AIDS death figures being listed as 'Deaths From African Swine Fever Virus?' long after the story had ceased to be viable. *Native* repeatedly attempted to make a connection between AIDS and the atrociously unethical experiment in Tuskegee where black people with syphilis were left untreated for forty years so the progress of the disease could be charted.

Of course, it is easier to dismiss conspiracy theories out of hand than to do the work which would substantiate or undermine them. The stories of Watergate and 'Irangate' tell us that some conspiracy theories won't go away because they describe real conspiracies.

Chuck Ortleb is aggressive and intense, stocky and virile, the sort of man who, if he were straight, would have women falling for him and other men wondering what they saw in him.

I remember sitting opposite him on the evening before we were planning to film an interview with him, and he was rattling away about the involvement of the CIA or the FBI or some other intelligence agency in the HIV story. I thought: 'We cannot have this wild-eyed lunatic talking like this on television. If he says this sort of thing to people in their own living rooms he will destroy the case for the alternatives to HIV. If he's on the team, people won't believe anyone.' Yet the next day when we set up to film here was a calm and urbane middle-aged man in a large and well-run newspaper office making considered statements about the irresponsibility of some research scientists.

But why had he always rejected HIV as the cause of AIDS?

I don't know that we've always rejected it. We've given it a lot of coverage. We've said it might be the cause of AIDS, we've also said it might not be the cause of AIDS. We're concerned about scientists who say it absolutely is the cause of AIDS, because science should never be that sure of itself.

We believe that both science and the publications that cover science should be very open minded, open to a spirit of inquiry. Something's very odd about AIDS. People are so emotional about their ideas and they don't want to hear new ideas about AIDS, there's something rotten about that.

After living through this epidemic, I trust scientists a little bit less than the average person.

Was Ortleb acting the first time, or the second, or both?

The criticism of Robert Gallo in the *Native* is particularly pungent. There would be no point in attempting to repeat such criticisms here; they would be removed on grounds of defamation long before publication. The challenge the *Native* presents is rather like that of John Wilkes who, when asked by a Frenchman 'How far does freedom of the press extend in your country?' answered, 'I don't know, I'm trying to find out.'

The great achievement of the *New York Native* is to have, alone among publications, maintained a spirit of inquiry. When everyone else toed the line and digested the material the press offices gave them, the *Native* asked questions, refused to accept contradictions. Latecomers like myself and all the other journalists who slowly realised there was a story in HIV which had not hit the mainstream, had to go to the *Native* for background because they were the only people who had done that work. They may have been wrong in some or even all of their campaigns but at least they had always acted like journalists.

The political undercurrent

The achievements of the nineteen-sixties, consolidated in the seventies, were changes in social structures to accommodate the changes which were occurring in personal behaviour. They were all civil rights victories: about the rights of women, of black people and of minorities. What would have been the response had a sample of the population been asked in 1959 if we would ever see cities run by black politicians, nations run by women politicians?

Related to this change, and an integral part of the fabric of liberal societies, was sexual freedom. The proposition that sexual freedom was an essential component of political freedom was the ball which the homosexual community picked up and ran with. It rapidly became accepted social doctrine that a society should not legislate about what adults can do with their bodies and that such legislation as did exist should be dismantled.

Sexual liberation occurred with astonishing rapidity, particularly after 1967 and the 'summer of love'. In England the three major reforms came in that year or the first months of the next. Homosexual acts in private were legalised for those over twenty-one. This was still five years higher than the age of consent for heterosexuals but at least it freed most men from legal attack.

Abortion was legalised, effectively giving women the right to control their own fertility. Free abortion and the right-wing attempts to limit or stop it became the central campaign of the women's movement, which relied for a good deal of its campaigning zeal on lesbians.

Censorship of the theatre was lifted. This may seem as if it would affect only a small number of people but in fact the theatre is queen of the arts in rather the same way that mathematics is said to be queen of the sciences. Theatrical conventions and preoccupations influence the other verbal arts and, with particular relevance for the second half of the twentieth century, cinema and television. The writers, actors, set designers, directors who crossed from one form to another ensured progress in the theatre meant progress in every medium.

The homosexuals were the storm troopers of sexual liberation. They went further and faster in sexual practice, as a group, than any but the most blessed of the heterosexual community. Probably only rock stars and groupies, over a short period of fame, could enjoy the level of sex which any young homosexual in a major city could have. When AIDS came it was greeted with undisguised glee by the right wing. 'The sexual revolution has begun to devour its own children,' wrote Patrick Buchanan in a syndicated column.

Buchanan, a former speech writer for Richard Nixon, had seen perfectly well what sexual freedom did for the values he believed in. It was time to go for the attack.

Buchanan said homosexuals should not be allowed to handle food or to work with children. Weakened and disunited by AIDS in May 1983 when Buchanan was writing, they also found themselves with few friends. The facts about the transmission of AIDS were not sufficiently widely known for Buchanan's beliefs about the casual transmission of AIDS to be understood for the nonsense they were. Homosexuals were fighting among themselves about the bathhouse closures. The most liberal of sexual campaigners might well lick their lips and look the other way if they were being asked to go to the barricades for the right of men to fuck each other to death.

The homosexuals had been separated off and attacked at their weakest. The victims were being seen as the perpetrators.

'AIDS is going to be the big human rights issue of the nineteen-nineties,' said Britain's gay rights leader Peter Tatchell. 'There is police harassment of gays and gay clubs in the provinces here; South Korea has just built a new half million pound detention centre; there are death squads in Brazil, people killing gays; nearly thirty countries have some form of travel restriction for people with HIV or AIDS.'

Christopher Monckton, a former adviser to Margaret Thatcher, has written *The AIDS Report* for circulation in right-wing circles. It demands annual blood tests for the entire population aged from thirteen to sixty-five and warns: 'Quarantining of AIDS carriers might be necessary.'

Brian Lantz and the Proposition 64 lobby in California in 1986 nearly achieved just that. His organisation, associated with the extreme right-wing LaRouche Democratic Campaign, achieved a referendum vote in 1986 to forbid anyone who tested positive for HIV antibodies from being 'allowed to work in or attend a public or private school in the state of California, nor would they be allowed to work in commercial food-handling establishments.' 'Quarantine' in camps would be the answer for those who refused to obey. It was defeated by only two to one.

Bavaria, not always remarkable for its liberalism, has since May 1987 permitted compulsory blood testing of suspected carriers and their quarantine if they are antibody-positive.

It is in these actions – sporadic and vicious but gaining in significance – where it is clear what damage the confusion of HIV antibodies with AIDS has done. Alleged public health measures could be used for the imprisonment of homosexuals and others the state finds undesirable. The public will not protest because, after all, aren't they being protected by these judicious measures?

It should not be thought that the persecution of homosexuals, with or without HIV antibodies, is the exclusive province of the political right. Homosexuals have traditionally been victims of authoritarians of all persuasions. At the international AIDS conference in London in January 1988 both the Soviet and Chinese delegates announced how a respect for family values and morality had kept their nations pure.

The fact that authoritarians have used the AIDS issue to increase their control over human lives does not mean they have conspired over it. There was no conspiracy, the authoritarians did not create AIDS, but when it did arrive, it perfectly suited the needs of those with a repressive and patriarchal state of mind.

By the mid-nineteen-eighties, with liberalism already in retreat, a single infection spread by sexual promiscuity and causing widespread death was the answer to the authoritarians' prayers. The involvement of heroin in the routes of transmission meant that sex and drugs, the rallying banners of sixties hedonism, were equally condemned. A medical message gained political currency fast because it confirmed views the politicians espoused. It may be true, of course, for all that, and HIV antibody positivity may be causally related to AIDS. But scientific fact was hardly the touchstone the politicians and columnists required to justify attacks on homosexuals.

The Fifth H

Very often what does not happen is as important as what does. In the world of scientific theorising this is particularly true. A prediction that a certain event will take place, based on known evidence and following a known theory, is one of the principal means of verifying or falsifying that theory.

It is very interesting therefore to remember the predictions being made on behalf of HIV in previous years. One prediction was that as AIDS is a sexually transmitted disease, transmissible by the acceptance of HIV infection alone, it followed that people who had the most sex would contract HIV first and develop AIDS first. These people who had a great deal of sex would act as the flag bearers for the disease. The people who had the most sex were prostitutes and they were earmarked as the next group to succumb, the 'bridging group' which would carry the disease from the original high-risk populations to the general population. To real people.

Newspaper journalists even had a catchy line to describe these new Typhoid Marys, they were the 'fifth H': hookers.

A number of journal articles and conferences pontificated on this new threat to mankind, including a *Lancet* article with Gallo as a co-author which was titled: 'Female Prostitutes: A Risk Group for Infection with Human T-Cell Lymphotropic Virus Type III'.

Randy Shilts in *And the Band Played On* records how a prostitute with AIDS was identified in the Tenderloin district of San Francisco on 3 January 1985. Immediately it was news: 'The uproar illuminated the profoundly heterosexual male bias that dominates the news business. After all, thousands of gay men had been infecting each other for years, but attempts to interest the news organisations to pressure the city for an aggressive AIDS education campaign had yielded minimal interest. A single female heterosexual prostitute, however, was a different matter. She might infect a heterosexual man. That was someone who mattered; that was news.'

The prostitute, thirty-four-year-old Silvana Strangis, was a heroin addict who had contracted AIDS from sharing infected needles. This was classically how prostitutes were expected to spread AIDS from the high-risk to the medium-risk population (the 'medium-risk' being contact with a prostitute), while the medium-risk would spread it to the low-risk – the monogamous wife at home. At least, that was the scenario: how one slip by a caring husband and father can bring the silent spectre of death to the previously happy hearthside. It was a compelling message, particularly in a nation like the US where the film *Fatal Attraction* enjoyed great success by representing the message metaphorically: AIDS can be seen as the woman who destroys a man's family life after an enjoyable one-night stand.

In fact prostitutes, and the clients of prostitutes, did not suffer such speedy retribution for their sins.

A series of studies in European cities, all published in the *Lancet*, confirmed that the danger to prostitutes was from intravenous drug use. While no Italian prostitutes in one particular study had lympha-denopathy syndrome, none were drug addicts. Of the drug addicts, forty-three per cent had it. In Athens, where prostitutes are licensed and none were said to be drug addicts, none had lymphadenopathy or AIDS. In the rue Saint-Denis in Paris intrepid researchers approached prostitutes and requested blood samples ('Quoi?') finding no evidence of AIDS.

Similarly in a West German study of 448 licensed prostitutes, none had lymphadenopathy or AIDS. With teutonic thoroughness the authors specified the practices of the prostitutes: 'thirteen per cent practice open-mouth kissing with clients. Seventy-four per cent occasionally to always masturbate clients, eighty per cent with condoms; sixty-three per cent occasionally to always perform oral sex, ninety per cent with condoms; ninety-two per cent occasionally to always have vaginal sex with clients, 97.5 per cent do this with condoms; and five per cent occasionally to always have rectal sex, 55.5 per cent with condoms.'

A study in London found a similar result – of fifty prostitutes none had any sign of AIDS. They came from a variety of milieux: obtaining their employment from the streets, escort agencies, advertisements, night clubs and brothels. All engaged in vaginal intercourse, forty-one having oral sex (thirty-five per cent swallowing semen) and nine had regular anal intercourse, three using condoms. This study noted that the AIDS scare itself may have influenced their behaviour towards sexual safety – thirty said all clients now wore condoms for all forms of penetrative intercourse. Nineteen had always insisted on this, even before AIDS.

Condom use can explain some of the low incidence of AIDS among European prostitutes, so can the lower incidence of drug addiction among European prostitutes than among those in American groups studied, in New York and Seattle, for example, where it is difficult to find a group of prostitutes to study which is 'uncontaminated' by drug use.

Another issue may be the general difficulty of contracting AIDS through vaginal or oral heterosexual encounters, particularly if those contacts took place only once with each partner. That is to say, a prostitute and a client are less likely to be enjoying lingering and repeated sexual acts over a period of years than a married couple are. Haemophiliac wives are therefore more likely to contract AIDS from an infected partner than prostitute suppliers of an infected client. Yet as we have seen, AIDS has not been such a serious problem among haemophiliac wives as was originally feared. This is not to diminish the individual suffering in those tragic cases where heterosexual infection has occurred this way.

An American study found the risk factors for AIDS in US women to be similar to those for prostitutes in the same areas. Using HIV antibodies as a test (this is an acceptable test even if HIV does not cause the disease as there is so often a correlation between the disease and the virus) it was found that 57.1 per cent of prostitutes in New Jersey, a major drug area, had antibodies. However, in Atlanta, Colorado Springs and Las Vegas the percentage was just over one to nil.

To put the 'heterosexual epidemic' into perspective, it is interesting to look at AIDS cases in the UK. Though there were 1598 reported AIDS cases to the middle of 1988, only ten of these were individuals who were infected heterosexually and had no evidence of having been infected abroad. There were six women and four men. Of these one was the wife of a haemophiliac; one was a female prostitute with many clients from the US; one was a woman who had sexual contact with several Africans; one was a woman who had contact with an intravenous drug user. One of the men had multiple sex partners, including contact with prostitutes and he shared a razor with a drug addict. I have no information on the other three men and two women. 'Sexual contact with Africans' is also a somewhat dubious 'risk factor', presumably it refers to the fact that AIDS appears to be transmitted by heterosexual sex more frequently in Africa than the West.

So in an advanced nation with a high standard of health care and no reason for under-reporting, an atmosphere as sexually liberated as almost anywhere else in the world, the heterosexual epidemic after seven years still amounted only to ten cases, most of them ascribable to contact with a high-risk individual.

The Far East

In a girlie bar in Bangkok's Patpong district a couple of girls with angelic faces and tiny breasts gyrate to pop music on a narrow stage. They are dressed only in briefs and in fluorescent stars which cover their nipples, as are the flock of other teenage girls who swarm the bar trying to attract the attention of the Western men who sit sipping beer and lapping up the attention. These men, ageing swingers from America, Germany, Britain and Australia, know they can have sex with girls here who wouldn't look twice at them back home. For the price of a round of drinks in their own country these men can do what they like all night with a girl who has been sold into a 'contract' with the bar by her land-slave father.

The men are generally professionals or skilled workers – the cost of a sex holiday in Thailand ensures that. Commonly around forty years old, the men bear the unmistakable mark of a good life gone to seed. Sitting alone or with girls who are little more than children, some of them wear gold medallions round their necks.

The advertisements coyly offer bars 'where love is waiting and Bangkok's most beautiful girls are eager to be your valentine tonight.

Let's fall in love!'. 'Talent scouts' have scoured the nation to find girls pretty and poor enough to work in the bars. The girls have a working life of, at the most, ten years. Suicide and drug addiction are threats to them, as is the danger of ending up in the unlucrative and far less glamorous Thai brothels, for local consumption only. A smart girl, however, is able to make sufficient money in a short working life to afford to buy a house or a shop in Thailand, thanks to the low cost of living there and the generosity of drunken and libidinous Westerners.

There is a danger of being too sanctimonious about cultures in which such blatant prostitution thrives, so it is as well to note that there are considerably less comfortable ways of earning a living than prostitution, in the West as well as in the Third World.

Prostitution really took off in Thailand when, in the early seventies, the Hong Kong government banned American servicemen from taking rest and recreation on its territory because of their rowdy behaviour. The men, who were taking part in the Vietnam war, were then sent to Thailand, which developed its small red light districts to cater for them. When the war ended the girlie bars remained and formed a lucrative source of revenue for the nation – people went to Thailand for a sex holiday; it was one of the major sex resorts in the world before AIDS was a problem and throughout the early years of AIDS.

There is male prostitution but it is far less significant. Only a few bars advertise, like the 'Golden Cock', that they offer 'gorgeous and young, all-in male entertainment'.

If prostitutes are major vectors for AIDS and heterosexual spread is easy, Thailand should have a major AIDS problem. This is particularly true considering one of the main attractions about visiting prostitutes there is the low rate of condom use.

In fact there is an extremely low rate of AIDS. In November 1987 there had been eleven AIDS cases. Eight men had died, four of them Westerners. Another three Thai men were in hospital.

It is possible, of course, that this is a lie and that there are far more cases but the government has covered them up or does not know about them. It is possible, but not likely. In terms of medical services, Thailand is often used as a model for the Third World. Undoubtedly there must be some people dying in squalor but anyone ill in a town, and towns are the centres of prostitution, would receive hospital attention. Additionally there are numerous private clinics offering tests for sexually transmitted diseases and public hospitals in Bangkok offer free testing for AIDS. The government tests large numbers of prostitutes in Bangkok and other cities and, as of July 1987, no female prostitute had even tested positive to HIV antibodies, so even this remote connection with AIDS was not apparent.

A perfidious government jealous of threats to its tourist revenues? Not really. Though hardly Western style, Thailand enjoys a democracy with a vigorous opposition which would take the usual delight in embarrassing their political opponents. Thailand also has a free press which, far from overlooking prostitution, makes it a current topic of debate. Items range from the gossip column noting that German women on holiday in Penang are enraging the local girls by doing a little freelance prostitution, to criticisms of police corruption in the editorials. This last was a reference to a raid on a brothel where the *Bangkok Post* remarked at the efficiency of the police in managing to arrest so many prostitutes but expressed surprise at their inability to arrest even one of the pimps. The 'free press' in Britain has never, to my knowledge, made such a comment, though the appearance in London courts of prostitutes is a daily occurrence, while pimps never appear.

Chantawipa Apisook of Empower, a group campaigning for AIDS awareness, criticises the Thai government, saying 'The government has no policy on AIDS. It is trying to control the media – otherwise the tourists won't come.' Representatives of AIDS pressure groups will always say resources are insufficient – as will representatives of every other pressure group about their cause. Generally it has taken some deaths to shake governments into action. The deaths took a long time in coming in Thailand. The Thai government and the US overseas aid agency USAID are jointly spending $7.5 million until 1992 on mass education about AIDS.

There will doubtless be a homosexual epidemic of AIDS in Thailand and in other South-east Asian countries like South Korea which put its number of cases at eleven at the end of 1987. There will probably be a very limited drug epidemic because needles are easily available, reducing the need for sharing, and there is a tradition of smoking opiates in the Far East which may be as addictive as intravenous use but is far less dangerous. There is no evidence to suggest the imminence of a heterosexual epidemic.

If an assertion is made that an event will occur, that prostitutes are going to suffer an AIDS epidemic, for example, it is up to those who believe in such an assertion to prove it, not up to those who disagree to demonstrate it untrue. There has as yet been no epidemic among prostitutes independent of intravenous drug use among them. Even among these women, taking the New York junkies as a model, there does not seem to have been an epidemic among their clients. 'Wait and see', say those who believe prostitute junkies are the angels who bring the message of death to the heterosexual world. But wait how long? The New York City Department of Health records deaths among intravenous drug users from AIDS as early as 1981, with suggestions that there were such deaths prior to 1979. The epidemic is taking its time.

As for prostitutes who are not intravenous drug users, they seem to be in no more danger – and therefore their clients share this – than other women in similar environments. This is a conundrum which only time will unravel. Greater care among clients and increased use of condoms may well have made a difference – but all over the world? And if, as we are always told by HIV supporters, the virus takes years before it becomes lethal, why are we not now seeing the AIDS cases among prostitutes who were failing to take precautions before there was an awareness of the danger of AIDS?

Prostitutes were, of course, well advised to use condoms. The danger of the whole range of sexually transmitted diseases is so great, AIDS should make no difference to the precautions prostitutes and their clients should always have taken.

Roy Anderson of the Department of Applied Biology at Imperial College in London explains the absence of a heterosexual epidemic by reference to the different rate of sexual contacts enjoyed by homosexuals and heterosexuals. Referring to studies which suggest homosexuals have twenty to twenty-five partners to every one–two in heterosexuals, he remarks:

> There is a roughly twenty-fold difference in the rate of partner change and in the absence of any other information, that magnitude of difference is likely to mean the epidemic will be moving and developing at a much lower timescale in the heterosexual community.
>
> If we're thinking in the homosexual community of a timescale of somewhere about ten to fifteen years we are probably thinking in the heterosexual community of a timescale in the maximum instance of twenty, thirty or more years.

Maybe so. But this is getting very far indeed from the model of HIV which says one dose is like being 'hit by a truck', the 'bang, bang, you're dead' image of a killer virus.

Six

Syphilis

'WHAT DO YOU do for a living?'

'I'm in death with dignity.'

The medical party joke rang in Stephen Caiazza's ears as his pitiably thin patient in the checked shirt and jeans closed the door behind him. He wore his shirt collar up in an attempt to hide the big Kaposi's sarcoma lesion on his neck but nothing could disguise the pale, waxy appearance of the AIDS victim.

Stephen Caiazza should have been at his strongest and most successful. A good-looking young doctor with a practice on Manhattan's Fifth Avenue, he was what everyone else would describe as a success. To himself he was a bitter failure. The patient he had just seen was going to die, so was the patient he saw before that, so was the one he saw before that. They hardly had three years' life left between them. This was the doom of youth, a carnage of young men unknown except in wartime.

Stephen had always wanted to be a doctor from the time he was a little boy. One of his earliest memories was going to the doctor with his mother and gaining a lasting impression of the power of medicine. 'I was so impressed by this man, that by the laying on of hands he could make sick people better, or so it seemed to me.'

He went to the New York School of Medicine and qualified as a doctor, then worked in private hospitals for a year to pay off the debts he had built up as a medical student. He hated working in a place where the bottom line was the bottom line – the credit line. He worked in a hospital which had the highest RPPD – Revenue Per Patient Day – in the area. That meant staff at that hospital were able to do more tests on patients and prescribe more drugs for them, thus pushing up the amount each patient was charged per day. It made money, but it wasn't medicine.

As soon as he could he left and set up his own private practice. The time was 1982 and the mysterious disease affecting homosexual men was still being called Gay Related Immune Deficiency Syndrome – GRIDS.

For four years he and his colleagues faced this plague with deepening despair as patients weakened and died in the most horrifying circumstances.

It was devastating. Our motivation was all directed to being healers, here we were just helping people to die. Some of my colleagues would try to create self-help groups but of course the people who were being helped would die. That's when we used to say: 'I'm in the death with dignity business.'

I was part of a big behind-the-scenes campaign to get AZT released, it was a drug we thought could do some limited good for AIDS patients, maybe it would do more than that. We had put pressure on the Food and Drug Administration to allow it to be released without all the required data because of the urgency of the AIDS situation and the early promise of the drug. The FDA relaxed some of its guidelines and we were pleased about that. It seemed like progress.

In fact the great breakthrough of Stephen Caiazza's life had already occurred, he just hadn't realised it. It was another of those cases where the thing which did not happen was more important than the thing which did. He was hardly seeing any cases of syphilis. He said:

While there was an exponential increase in AIDS, I was only getting one or two cases of syphilis per year. I had one of the biggest gay practices in Manhattan and I thought it strange that syphilis was going away while AIDS was increasing, especially as they are both transmitted in the same way.

In addition, a few of my patients with full-blown AIDS would sometimes come up with a positive VDRL (Venereal Disease Research Laboratory) or some other serological result indicating infection with syphilis. Those patients I treated in the standard way for syphilis, with penicillin, and their AIDS got better. This was just a coincidence, I thought, something I wasn't looking for.

When a couple of patients had presented with unusual lesions in the throat and the gall bladder, he treated them for syphilis. The lesions disappeared. He began to suspect there was some confusion between AIDS and syphilis but this could be just interference at the testing stage – antibodies in the blood signalling the presence of one or another pathogen could be confusing the tests, a better test would give a more definite result. Stephen did not herald this as a great discovery; after all, syphilis has been around for a long time. He just chatted to his colleagues about it.

One day in September 1986 he was at home feeling tired and miserable when the telephone rang. It was Joan McKenna, a scientist from California who had been working with AIDS patients and the 'worried well', generally helping them to make lifestyle changes and 'get their immune system back into shape'. She too had noticed the link with syphilis.

'I understand you're interested in the role of syphilis in AIDS,' she said.

'Yes.'

'Have you heard of Dr Dierig in Augsburg?'

'I've never heard of Augsburg, let alone Dr Dierig.'

She explained the work of the German doctor and within forty-eight hours he was on the plane to Augsburg with the notes on his patients. Stephen Caiazza, Klaus-Uwe Dierig and Urban Waldthaler sat in a bar and compared notes. The Germans not only believed syphilis could be confused with AIDS, in many if not all cases they thought syphilis *was* AIDS.

So what was syphilis?

The Great Pox, so called to distinguish it from smallpox, spread through Europe, Asia and as far as China shortly after Christopher Columbus returned from Haiti in 1493.

The Columbian theory of its origin is that syphilis was brought from Haiti by Columbus' crew. In support of this is the Barcelona physician R. de Isla who recorded 'an illness not seen nor recorded nor heard of previously in Barcelona', which was present in the sailors. The fact that the crew called it 'Indian measles' implies they associated it with the places they had visited on the voyage.

It is characteristic of the popular nomenclature of sexually transmitted diseases, it should be said, to be attributed to aliens. The Italians called syphilis the French malady, the French called it the Spanish complaint, continental Europe called it the English pox. It became known as Naples sickness after the siege of Naples in 1493 when mercenary armies from all over Europe met and, presumably, had adequate time for leisure while the long process of besieging or being besieged took place. Ill health stopped the siege and the mercenaries dispersed throughout the known world.

Syphilis was extremely virulent at this time, many dying within weeks of infection. This strongly suggests a new disease to which the host population had had no time to build up an immunity.

Syphilis spread through Europe, Asia including India and in 1505 was recorded in Canton, China. Thus, according to the Columbian theory, in twelve years syphilis had spanned the known world from the sexual contacts of Columbus and a crew of forty-four men. Prodigious activity.

An alternative theory, the African or Unitarian theory, takes into account earlier reports of a disease which may have been syphilis. There are descriptions of a disease which may have been syphilis in ancient Chinese, Indian, Hebrew and Greek writings and prehistoric bones show some evidence of syphilis.

This theory suggests syphilis has always been with humans but has evolved along with its host's movements and behaviour patterns. The claim is that there was a bacterial ancestor to all the syphilis-like diseases which currently infect humans. Thus yaws, endemic (child-hood) syphilis, venereal syphilis, bejel, pinta and other diseases of a similar type all started in the mists of time as a single disease, something like yaws, somewhere in Africa. As prehistoric people moved from tropical Africa towards the north (the Sahara), the environment changed from the moist, humid rain forest to dry and cooler areas in North Africa and Asia. The bacteria which infected, then, the whole of the body, found the new environment not conducive to continued existence and retreated to the warm, moist parts of the body – the genitals, mouth, anus.

This produced endemic syphilis, as did the move to crowded and unsanitary town life. Until recent mass campaigns, endemic syphilis affected most children born in the villages of the North African deserts, the plains of Asia and the steppes of Eastern Europe. These were the last areas to see widespread endemic syphilis which had in earlier centuries affected Yugoslavia, Scotland, Scandinavia and Ireland.

Other means of transition from yaws to endemic to venereal syphilis occurred when cities evolved and the crowded conditions demanded greater sanitation than had been the case in towns and villages. In the cities of China, Egypt and Greece, to cite the earliest, the cleanliness ensured by sewerage systems and clean water supplies was another threat to the bacteria. They retreated further into their new home of the sexual organs.

The slave trade has also been suggested as a means of the syphilis bacteria developing from the yaws bacteria. 100 million slaves were, it is estimated, taken from Africa over the centuries to serve the

Egyptians, Greeks, Romans, Persians, Spanish, Portuguese, British and Americans. When they were sent to drier and colder countries yaws could develop into endemic then venereal syphilis.

The advantage of the African theory is that it allows for the evolution of what is certainly a fast replicating bacteria in millions of people over thousands of years. It is more elegant as a theory than the idea that a single shipload of sailors infected the world. The Columbian theory also doesn't tell us where syphilis came from or how it could be so closely related to diseases like yaws and pinta which are endemic to Africa. How did the Haitians get it?

Unfortunately the present tools of history and science are unable to answer questions of the origin of syphilis, despite our familiarity with it. This does not augur well for the future of theories of the origin of AIDS. The syphilis question may be answered when it is possible to propagate it in a laboratory culture. At the moment it is as well simply to note that an informed body of opinion supports the theory that syphilis will alter to adapt to its conditions.

Syphilis in history

Syphilis tore through Europe and Asia in the sixteenth century. One estimate is that it reduced the population of Europe by between a sixth and a third. Public health laws, particularly in seaports where the disease was known to flourish first, attempted to control prostitutes and quarantine those infected with the disease.

Another public health measure was the writing of an allegorical poem by one Girolamo Fracastoro of Verona who described Syphilus, a swineherd, who was smitten by the disease when he refused to make a sacrifice to Apollo. From him the Great Pox got its modern name. The poem was called *Syphilis sive morbus Gallicus* – Syphilis, or, the French Disease.

For centuries mercury was the only even mildly effective remedy, though some physicians felt the later ravages of the disease might well be due to mercury poisoning rather than syphilis.

Progress was also delayed by a belief that gonorrhoea and syphilis were the same disease. Syphilis can be virtually symptomless in the early stages but is always devastating in the end. Gonorrhoea causes acute pain on urination early in the infection which then subsides. Alexander Pope celebrated: 'Time that at last matures a clap to pox.'

This mistaken idea gave rise to one of the most heroic episodes in the history of medicine when John Hunter in 1767 inoculated himself with pus from the genitals of a patient suffering from gonorrhoea. When he developed both gonorrhoea and syphilis, it was a proof they were the same, so he thought. In fact the patient had both gonorrhoea and syphilis, proof that dedication and courage will not alone produce the correct result. Some commentators have wondered whether he inoculated himself or a patient.

By the first decade of the seventeenth century the virulent, swiftly fatal form of syphilis gave way to the smouldering endemic form which may well have played its part in the AIDS epidemic.

The progress towards the elimination of syphilis in this century gives a far more realistic picture of how diseases are understood and, hopefully, mastered, than the *Boy's Own* image of microbe hunters. In ripping yarns of this type a boy sees a family member die of an incurable illness, he swears to become a doctor and find a cure. Through many disadvantages and setbacks his determination wins through – he discovers the microbe which causes the disease and develops a vaccine to cure it. Then he goes to Stockholm to collect his Nobel Prize.

That is a good story, but bad history. It actually happens more like this: Elie Metchnikoff and Pierre Roux in 1903 managed to inoculate a laboratory animal with syphilis; this led to lab work which allowed Fritz Schaudinn and Erich Hoffman to isolate the spiral-shaped bacteria now known as Treponema pallidum. Because they had the animal model it was possible to prove the bacteria actually caused the disease – they could give it to the animal, cause the disease, extract it from that animal and put it in another one and cause the disease again.

The causal agent for syphilis had been sought for as long as bacteriology had existed and repeatedly wrongly identified. One observer noted drily: 'One hundred and twenty-five causes of syphilis have been established during the last twenty-five years.'

August von Wassermann in 1910 devised a test for syphilis. It was not always successful but at least now there was a test. It was possible now to tell who had syphilis, even if the disease was in a latent form, with reasonable accuracy for the period.

Paul Ehrlich tried different preparations of arsenic on syphilis and finally, in 1910, the 606th compound tested was successful. Salvarsan, as it was called, was the first effective drug against syphilis. The bacteria was able, if it had been given an insufficient dose, to develop an immunity to Salvarsan but it was the first scientifically developed drug despite its limitations.

In a bold experiment in 1917 Julius Wagner-Jauregg inoculated a patient with advanced neurosyphilis with a strain of malaria, which brought some relief as Salvarsan could not in this advanced condition.

Sir Alexander Fleming's discovery of penicillin in 1928 did not contribute to the treatment of syphilis until Howard Florey and Ernst Chain investigated and purified it in 1940. It was first used to treat syphilis in the US in 1943 with dramatic results.

An accurate test for syphilis continued to elude researchers. Nelson and Mayer in 1949 devised the Treponema pallidum immobilisation test which was able to test for antibodies against syphilis. It is so complex and expensive, it is now obsolete and more recently developed but less reliable tests are used. The failure of science to produce a simple but effective test for syphilis is central to the world-wide problem of untreated or poorly treated syphilis and to the contribution syphilis has made to the AIDS epidemic.

A lurking disease

In earlier centuries the problem of syphilis was the ravages of its later phases. For the last half of the twentieth century the problem is the respite it gives a sufferer: the latency period of lurking disease.

There are four periods of syphilis: primary, secondary, latent and tertiary.

Primary syphilis

This is evident from nine days to three months after sex with an infected person. The primary sore or chancre appears at the spot where the Treponema pallidum bored its way into the body. In men this is on the glans penis, the shaft or the scrotum or in the case of passive homosexuals in or around the anus. It can therefore easily be missed.

In women it appears on the cervix, the inner vaginal walls or the vaginal lips. It frequently goes unnoticed in women.

The open sore which may be covered by a yellow or grey scab will heal by itself within one to five weeks of its appearance. The disease continues to develop, however, and is still highly infectious.

Secondary syphilis

This stage is characterised by a skin rash – small round, rose-pink spots on the shoulders, upper arms, chest, back and stomach. After a few weeks or days the spots become brownish and fade.

Another manifestation of the rash is red bumps becoming brown (on white skin) all over the body including the palms and soles of the feet. On black skin the bumps are greyish blue.

Mucous patches in the throat are one of the ways the syphilitic rash may present.

It is in the phase of secondary syphilis that the disease earns its name as 'The Great Masquerader' and which had led to generations of doctors being brought up on the dictum of Sir William Osler that: 'He who understands syphilis understands medicine.'

In common with AIDS, syphilis presents as a series of other conditions do. A characteristic is lymphadenopathy – the swollen lymph glands which are common in patients with the early stages of AIDS, with people who have been infected with cytomegalo (the 'passenger or driver?') virus and Epstein-Barr virus causing the 'kissing disease' – glandular fever.

Patients will suffer from headaches, loss of appetite with attendant weight loss, night sweats, insomnia, pain in bones and joints, fever. Some patients have a swollen liver or spleen, high blood pressure, kidney disease.

Syphilis in this stage is most frequently confused with iritis (inflammation of the iris); psoriasis and other skin diseases; cancer; nephritis (inflammation of the kidney); dementia; lymphomas (disorders of the lymphatic system) and adverse drug reactions.

There are clinical manifestations, in addition to the rash which may be mild and be overlooked, in about half the infected people. Syphilis is at its most dangerous in its secondary stage and can spread most rapidly, particularly, of course, from those who have no symptoms.

This stage may last up to two years, though generally it disappears within three months. Above twenty-five per cent of people show a relapse into the secondary phase after moving on to the third, latent phase.

Latent syphilis

This is that period when the disease is completely hidden. About a third of people live the rest of their lives with no further problems from the disease, though the characteristic of syphilis to imitate other diseases means that the patient may die from 'heart disease', for example, when in fact the spirochete has invaded the heart and attacked the aorta or aortic valve. Fifteen or more years may pass when the disease is not apparent. Blood tests may be negative for syphilis. It is not infectious except in that a pregnant woman can pass it on to her child *in utero* – another strong similarity with AIDS.

To demonstrate the ease with which syphilis can be undiagnosed or misdiagnosed: a survey of thirty-four patients with secondary syphilis treated in a Detroit public health clinic found only fourteen of the physicians who had seen them had given syphilis as the primary diagnosis. Five others had included it in the differential diagnosis.

In a screening of 1820 patients over fifty-five attending a hospital in Sheffield, England, forty-six patients had evidence of syphilis. Specifically in relation to the age of the patients, the authors noted that at the beginning of the century, the probability of dying directly as a result of untreated syphilis was seventeen per cent: 'The results suggest that there remains a large group of patients with undiagnosed syphilis that will only be picked up by routine screening.'

Tertiary syphilis

This is the horror familiar to readers of history and literature. Huge destructive ulcers affect the face, legs, upper trunk and scalp. These are the cutaneous (skin) gumma.

The even more distressing mucosal gumma affect the nose and mouth, destroying mucosal tissue – effectively an eating away of the mouth and nose. The nose can take on a trumpet shape, opening out with a hole in the centre.

Thickening of the bones and inflammation of bony tissue causes crippling pain.

Many other organs of the body are involved in the disease if untreated: the liver, eyes, stomach, lungs and testes.

Gumma infection of the brain leads to pain and mental disturbance which eventually resembles paralysis, in that patients become unable to carry out basic motor functions, they don't have sufficient brain cells to work out what they want to do, a condition called 'walnut brain' on autopsy. This condition, general paresis, was once a major cause of patients being sent to mental hospitals. George Csonka remarks: 'The old aphorism that "everyone suffers in general paresis but not the patient" is still true. The patient has no insight into his condition and often has a vacant expression or a fatuous smile. A degree of inappropriate boastful euphoria is present in a minority of patients but more common is progressive dementia until a state is reached where a patient is unable to feed himself, is incontinent and bedridden, and leads a vegetative existence.'

Lightning pain in the legs or feet herald tabes dorsalis (wasting of the back). Numbness in walking and gastric problems give way to an inability to walk, reflex failure, muscle weakness, impotence and double incontinence.

Csonka remarks that there is some evidence that syphilis is becoming milder and less typical. There has been the virtual disappearance of the gumma and a decline in neurosyphilis. This is perhaps because of widespread antibiotic use and perhaps because the disease was tending to become 'milder' even before the antibiotic era.

Stephen Caiazza speaks almost respectfully of the disease for its persistence and adaptability: 'Throughout history this disease, the great masquerader, has proven itself able to do anything it wants. In the fifteenth century, when Western Europe first became familiar with syphilis, it was a great plague that wiped out twenty-five per cent to a third of the population. Later on we reached a natural balance with the organism. Today we are seeing a resurgence of the great masquerader in another form.'

Just how far even tertiary syphilis can masquerade was demonstrated by a study of 241 patients with neurosyphilis at the Medical College of Virginia from July 1965 to July 1970. Nearly half the patients (47.8 per cent) had never been diagnosed for any kind of syphilis, let alone tertiary neurosyphilis.

The syphilis tests

There are at least twelve tests for syphilis in current use – the proliferation of different types of tests in itself suggests their limitations – no test is so good it has beaten the opposition.

The problem of undiagnosed syphilis is partly because the disease 'hides' in its latent phase and is not seen at all; partly because it 'masquerades' as other diseases and partly because of the limitations of the tests even when they are performed. One text book says:

A 'false negative' serological test can occur when the infection is too recent to have triggered the production of antibodies. A negative result can also occur if the disease is in a latent or inactive phase or if the patient's immune system is not functioning normally. If treatment of syphilis had been started before the test, the patient's blood could be temporarily non-reactive. Since alcohol interferes with and decreases the intensity of a reaction, it should be considered as a possible cause of a negative result.

The most common tests are the Venereal Disease Research Laboratory (VDRL) and the rapid plasma reagin (RPR) tests.

Stephen Caiazza noticed that his patients usually tested negative when these tests were used but found when the most sophisticated fluorescent treponomal antibody absorbed test (FTA-ABS) was used, almost all his AIDS patients tested positive for syphilis. Overnight, his AIDS patients became syphilis patients.

Comparing clinical successes with the German workers was exciting but they needed stronger scientific data. Stephen Caiazza had been storing sera from his patients; he packed twenty samples of it in dry ice and sent it to Germany for tests, deliberately choosing a majority of cases who had tested negative for syphilis in the past. With the most sophisticated tests, they were positive.

It was no surprise that there should be a great deal of syphilis in the homosexual community. To quote directly from Harris Coulter's book *AIDS and Syphilis – the Hidden Link*: 'In the United States today the homosexual male is fourteen times more likely to have had syphilis than the heterosexual male; seventy-five per cent of syphilis cases are in males, of whom half are either bisexual or homosexual.'

George Csonka noted that the European figures were similar: the syphilis figures were rising in the nineteen-seventies and homosexual men were taking 'more than their share' of the figures: in 1971 homosexual males accounted for fifty per cent of early syphilis, in 1980 it was fifty-eight per cent. Syphilis was increasingly not only a male but a homosexual male disease.

Stephen Caiazza and his colleagues began gathering information. He found that all the clinical signs and symptoms associated with AIDS have also been described in syphilis. If an AIDS patient could have been transported back to 1900 any venereologist would have diagnosed a syphilitic. Doctors trained after World War Two, when syphilis was treatable almost to the point of its disappearance, had simply never learned how important it was to exclude syphilis in a diagnosis. It was still all there in the medical textbooks.

The skin lesions in syphilis are indistinguishable from those in Kaposi's sarcoma. Indeed, there may be a closer relationship: Moriz Kaposi first described the skin condition which bears his name at the dermatology clinic in Vienna, in a group of syphilitic patients.

The lung parasite Pneumocystis carinii which causes Pneumocystis carinii pneumonia, the rapidly fatal disease in AIDS patients, can easily be confused with 'white lung' pneumonia in syphilis. Another interesting connection involves animal work: two monkeys inoculated with Treponema pallidum and put in a cage with healthy monkeys, infected all the healthy monkeys. After forty-four months all the monkeys had died of Pneumocystis carinii pneumonia.

As will be remembered, Pneumocystis carinii pneumonia was long known to infect those with weakened immune systems. One of the chief characteristics of syphilis is immune suppression.

The treatment of syphilis

The treatment of syphilis prescribed by the Centers for Disease Control in the USA is one shot of benzathine penicillin (2.4 million units). At this point the level of antibodies to the treponemes (the 'titre') falls. The CDC manual on syphilis notes: 'Titres should become non-reactive in six to twelve months following treatment for primary syphilis, and twelve to eighteen months following treatment for secondary syphilis.

'Treatment of a late latent or late infection usually has little or no effect on the titre.

'Titres tend to become lower with time but frequently remain reactive in low titre.'

For late or latent syphilis the CDC prescribes a further two doses of benzathine penicillin. Many people are stuck with high antibody titres; they are referred to as 'serofast', but because they have had the treatment they are considered to have been cured. As Craig Johnson writes in the *New York Native*: 'I find it especially curious that when someone is seropositive for the antibody to HIV, the so-called "AIDS virus", he's presumed to be a "carrier", but when he's seropositive for the antibodies to syphilis, he's presumed to be cured.'

Those who maintain there has been a reservoir of untreated syphilis cases contributing to the AIDS epidemic say this has occurred for two main reasons. Firstly the doses given are too low – Stephen Caiazza and his colleagues recommend 40 million units as compared to the CDC's 2.4 million. In addition to not curing the disease, but only driving it into a latent form, this treatment allows the treponemes to develop an immunity to penicillin. This immunity may, incidentally, have some relationship to the virulence and speed of the disease from which AIDS patients suffer. Penicillin itself can be immunosuppressive, as can be the many other antibiotics which may be taken by a person suffering from diarrhoea because of gut infections; chronic sore throat; gonorrhoea and other illnesses characteristic of the 'fast track' lifestyle.

The second reason for the under-treatment of syphilis is related to the lifestyle of the spirochete Treponema pallidum itself. It can be destroyed by penicillin only when it is actively replicating itself. In the beginning, when a person is first infected, it takes thirty-three hours for the spirochete to divide.

The longer a person has the spirochete, the longer the dividing time. If a person has syphilis for months or even a year or so before it is suspected, the dividing time could be 120 to 240 days.

This means syphilis must be treated for a long time, far longer than had previously been thought necessary, in order for the organism to be eradicated at its vulnerable time.

A further problem of dealing with this adaptable spirochete is that it 'hides' out of reach of the usual treatment.

The benzathine penicillin used today cannot penetrate the blood–brain barrier – the barrier separating the blood from the brain which is permeable by water, oxygen, carbon dioxide and some other substances such as glucose, alcohol and general anaesthetics. Basically, the benzathine penicillin molecules are too big to pass through the barrier.

This is only a problem because the Treponema pallidum make their way to the brain and eye and live there as a reservoir of infection. As Carol Berry and colleagues from the University of Washington School of Medicine reported in the *New England Journal of Medicine* as recently as 18 June 1987: 'The recommended therapeutic agent for primary, secondary and latent syphilis, benzathine penicillin, does not reach treponemicidal levels [that is, able to kill treponemes] within the cerebrospinal fluid, and concerns have been raised that current treatment regimens may be inadequate, particularly in patients who harbour spirochetes in their central nervous systems.'

The increasing appearance of 'AIDS dementia' is now being seen by some as neurosyphilis.

There are several reasons for the failure of the US authorities (and all the other national public health authorities who follow CDC advice) to deal adequately with latent syphilis. The disease takes a long time to develop, for example, and is often confused with other diseases as has been mentioned. This means few doctors will have followed patients through from inadequate treatment to recurrence of the disease. This is particularly true because of the mobility of the population in the US, including more especially those who enjoy a 'fast track' lifestyle.

Moreover, syphilis patients' relapses could be confused with re-infection, the doctors presuming that people who had once suffered infection with Treponema pallidum would continue with the sort of behaviour which might make them likely to become infected again.

Another reason for the inadequate treatment is also rooted in doctors' notions of how their patients will behave. One large dose of a drug which stays in the body for two weeks is, it is thought, the best type of treatment for patients who behave fecklessly and could not be expected to return for a repeat dose. British doctors have treated syphilis with at least one and often more repeat doses, week by week, with tests for antibodies in between, to ensure the treatment was effective.

World Health Organization recommendations are for a similar treatment to that of the US: a single dose but of only 1.8 million units.

The problem for effective treatment of syphilis is that aqueous penicillin, which will cross the blood–brain barrier can be administered only intravenously in a hospital. It is obviously impractical to put patients in hospital for twenty days to receive their forty million units of aqueous penicillin a day. Instead Caiazza treats them with high doses of benzathine penicillin 'to clear up the peripheral symptoms', then after three weeks he gives them doxycycline orally for several months because it does cross the blood–brain barrier.

The patients

Tom, a New York voice teacher, started with the familiar fevers, night sweats and fatigues in December 1986. Over the next few months he was feeling worse and was finally prescribed AZT, the drug which has been claimed to have had limited success in holding back AIDS. Then in August he had a recurrence of the Pneumocystis carinii pneumonia, almost always the fatal illness after repeated attacks. Tom had despaired of recovery. He had known enough AIDS patients to know what happened to them.

Then he saw Stephen Caiazza on a TV show and called him the next day. Tom said:

> His explanation tied in with what made sense to me. He took me off AZT right away and all other medication and started his penicillin therapy.
>
> I felt better immediately, on the first night with the penicillin shot I felt my head open up. It was like a relief from the pressure on my temples that I had experienced for over a year, even before I was diagnosed. It's been fine since that first night, and my energy has been boundless ever since.

Individual case histories cannot be used to 'prove' a theory of this nature, of course. Tom has only been treated for six months at time of writing. At best, it is possible to say an AIDS patient has had six months of sickness-free life, we cannot be sure about tomorrow. It is a better record than any other therapy, however.

At worst we have here a patient with syphilis who was misdiagnosed as having AIDS and mistakenly treated as if he had AIDS. Even this scenario shows Stephen Caiazza to be a rather good doctor. The former human skeletons in his waiting room are happy, healthy young men now.

Of course, there are too few patients and they have been involved for too short a period. Stephen Caiazza has been putting his theories into practice only since April 1987 and has been studying just over 125 patients. With one exception all are doing well. Time will tell.

Critics of his method might claim that with the vast doses of antibiotics he uses, he is simply aggressively treating the opportunistic infections and AIDS will resurface soon. There are two answers to this. The first is that if it is so easy to treat opportunistic infections and give AIDS patients a better life, why isn't everyone doing it? The other answer is : 'The drugs I am using don't fight the opportunistic infections which are most common. How would the use of penicillin explain the Kaposi's sarcoma that is going away? It's a skin cancer. I haven't written a prescription for medication for Pneumocystis in over a year, yet antibiotics won't get rid of the parasite that causes it. I'm writing less prescriptions for medication for thrush which is a fungus. Do all these have a bacterial cause?'

Problems with the syphilis hypothesis

There are several problems with the theory that AIDS is closely related to syphilis. Syphilis is a slow-burn disease. Why are the victims of AIDS getting sick with conditions which may well be symptomatic of syphilis but which do not normally occur in three years and then cause death?

This is where HIV comes in. Stephen Caiazza feels it may be playing an accelerating role:

> Spirochetes cause AIDS. HIV may be facilitating the work of the spirochetes but in terms of a causal role, no, HIV does not cause AIDS. The virus may be accordianising the forty or fifty years of a syphilitic infection into a few months or years.
>
> Bottom line, AIDS probably is syphilis. That's not quite accurate, but it is certainly the case that in an HIV-infected individual, if there is no syphilis there will be no clinical disease.

There is not a great problem in relating this theory to the major risk groups who comprise the vast majority of AIDS cases in the West: homosexuals certainly enjoyed a lifestyle which might predispose them to syphilis. They were also very unlikely ever to use condoms, which offer heterosexuals at least some protection. Haitians too might well have contracted syphilis sexually and the chances of effective treatment in Haiti would be remote. Heroin users would receive the disease on infected needles as they receive hepatitis B. Similarly transfusion-related cases would receive the infection in contaminated blood. Infection *in utero* of foetuses by their mothers is, of course, a hallmark of syphilis even in its latent phase.

The haemophiliacs are a real problem. Factor VIII, the only means by which most haemophiliac AIDS victims could have become infected, is an agent which can be filtered – this means nothing as large as a cell could get through. The spirochete which causes syphilis is as long as the height of a red blood cell. There is a suggestion that the spirochete could enter a 'pleomorphic' form, that is, it could change its shape while retaining its genetic material so it could reconstitute itself. This has not been observed before and is not likely. Perhaps it is not the spirochete itself which causes the disease but a parasite which lives on the spirochete and could penetrate the Factor VIII filter. Again, this is piling supposition on supposition. Stephen Caiazza does not hold to outlandish theories to explain haemophiliac cases; he simply says he does not know.

The other problem is the heterosexual population. If we have been inadequately treating syphilis for forty years and promiscuous heterosexual sex has been going on for at least that long, why haven't the heterosexuals got AIDS?

Stephen Caiazza said: 'There are some unfortunate sociologic truths about AIDS that we're going to have to admit to ourselves. One of these unpleasant truths is that in the major metropolitan areas the gay population has more sexual partners on average than the heterosexual population. You are playing a game of statistics, a game of Russian roulette. The gay population took that gun, put it to its head and simply pulled the trigger more often. The heterosexual population if it plays the same game, while it will take longer, will also win.'

But an epidemic of syphilis really is insufficient to explain the AIDS epidemic which started in so many places at roughly the same time. Syphilis could at best be a contributory factor which requires another factor or factors.

As Joe Sonnabend said: 'I don't think that syphilis is the cause of AIDS. I think that syphilis may well be a contributory factor in a situation where multiple factors do interact to produce the immune deficiency. Syphilis, certainly in its secondary stage is well known to have immunosuppressive effects.

'Amongst individuals who have AIDS and who have syphilis, an unusually high number of people, it is reasonable to suppose the syphilis contributes something.'

Research

Research is desperately needed on the connection between syphilis and AIDS. Obviously there is some connection. Stephen Caiazza and his colleagues have failed to interest research bodies in work on syphilis. They are not assisted in their efforts by the fact that there is almost certainly no money at the end of the research rainbow. If a more definite link is proved with syphilis, it will prove that cheap generic drugs can be used in AIDS – hardly the answer to the pharmaceutical industry's prayers. Stephen Caiazza jokes that if he had discovered a new strain of Treponema pallidum which could only be treated with expensive new medicines under licence to a drug company, he would have no trouble in raising funds.

The other problem with research on syphilis is that HIV has gobbled up all the research funds and all the researchers. An obsession with HIV alone has edged out other promising ideas. As Harris Coulter wrote: 'Researchers avid for Nobel prizes may be repelled by the prospect of having once again to tackle the intractable problem of syphilis instead of pursuing some glamorous new virus from an exotic African country.'

Stephen Caiazza is not the world's greatest research scientist and has never claimed to be. Stephen Caiazza is a caring physician who followed simple deductions based on his own clinical judgement of the condition of his own patients. He may be wrong or, more likely, only partially right. But at least he was looking where the disease is, in living patients co-existing with their environment.

Why do antibiotics work on some AIDS patients?

It may or may not be relevant that the various tests for the presence of Treponema pallidum cannot distinguish between other treponemes and this spirochete, which causes venereal syphilis, endemic syphilis and two other conditions called bejel and njovera. Other treponemes which cause disease are Treponema pertenue causing yaws and Treponema carateum causing pinta.

It is possible, therefore, that the symptoms of AIDS are actually caused by a spirochete which is not Treponema pallidum but another which causes a fast-acting syphilis. It is conceivable that people with multiple sexual partners could have incubated and reincubated a mutant form of spirochetes until a killer strain appeared. The tests would just show positive for a spirochete, they would not be specific. This is basically the ground plan for the 'Unitarian' model of the source of syphilis referred to earlier: other members of the Treponema family mutated to accommodate new human behaviour. This sort of suggestion is only susceptible to investigation by researchers going back to the patients, back to the patients' blood.

The question of what type of agent the AIDS microbe is has a central position in any question of treatment. Viruses are highly adaptable microbes which have no cell wall themselves. They have been described as bundles of genetic material wrapped in a protein coat. They have to combine with a cell in order to replicate. They are almost always far smaller in size than bacteria. Some of the common diseases they cause include chicken pox, measles and flu. Almost the only contribution of virology to public health has been the vaccination programme – strengthening human immunity against a possible viral infection. Almost no effective anti-viral drugs exist – the exception is acyclovir, a Wellcome drug which is effective in stopping a herpes outbreak from spreading (though not in preventing it starting) by halting viral replication. Viruses are, because of the difficulty of understanding them, at the forefront of scientific research. They require expensive equipment and sharp minds for their study and they also attract research funding.

The study of bacteria and bacterial diseases has gone into a decline from the pre-eminent period it enjoyed at the beginning of this century.

Most bacteria can be seen with an ordinary microscope. The discoveries of the bacteria which cause serious diseases were made many years ago, the Nobel Prizes have long since been awarded.

Most bacteria are treatable by the administration of antibiotics. There are specific antibiotics which attack specific bugs – metronidazole works against Giardia lamblia, which causes diarrhoea, for example, and others like the great penicillin itself are general killers of bacteria.

The Danes have done pioneering work on the treatment of AIDS patients with antibiotics. A thirty-eight-year-old homosexual AIDS patient reported to the dermatology department in the Finsen Institute in Copenhagen in October 1983. He had no history of recurrent infectious diseases but he had been treated for syphilis in 1978. The immediate cause of his distress was Kaposi's sarcoma: he had two large plaques on his right thigh and experience showed that these lesions were sure to increase over time. When the man was examined he was seen to have enlarged lymph nodes. Amus Poulsen looked at his patient and realised there was no hope. He could be made comfortable but he would be dead in two years. There being nothing to lose, he tried a drug he had recently heard spoken of at a scientific meeting. It was dapsone. He had heard of it before, of course, everyone had. Dapsone is specific to leprosy; it kills Mycobacterium leprae. Amus Poulsen treated his patient with dapsone and nothing else and after six weeks the Kaposi's sarcoma lesions had regressed and turned into brownish scars. What happened later to that patient is not recorded.

More thrilling was the work done by Vigo Faber and his colleagues at the University Hospital of Copenhagen in 1986. A fifty-eight-year-old man first presented to them with lethargy, fever and weight loss in 1984. He had generalised lymphadenopathy and HIV infection. He remained stable until 1986 when he got rapidly worse, suffering further weight loss and diarrhoea. He had inflammation of the stomach lining and the throat fungus Candida albicans (thrush). The bacteria which cause tuberculosis, Mycobacterium tuberculosis, was found and Vigo Faber decided to treat his patient with the drug fusidic acid. This is specific against the tuberculosis bacterium but little else, it was thought.

The patient got better. His fever went, he began to put on weight. In two weeks he was a changed man. He had been a living skeleton but he became a normal, healthy man and returned to work.

It must have been difficult to know what to do with this sort of case. Of course it must be reported so other patients could enjoy the benefit of it but to claim they had cured AIDS with an antibiotic would risk inviting the sort of reception Stephen Caiazza received. They did something very smart. They went to a member of the AIDS establishment and asked, all innocence: 'Could you give us some advice on the antiviral activity of this old antibiotic? It seems to inhibit the development of HIV.'

So an article went into the *Lancet* about the successful treatment of an AIDS patient with somewhat bogus material about what this old antibiotic is said to do to HIV in test tubes. Fusidic acid was used experimentally in the US and Canada. The patients received a promising drug, the HIV lobby was happy and the Danes got the thanks for it. Even if it does not realise its promise, the story of fusidic acid throws an interesting light on the way AIDS research must be presented in order to be treated seriously. Viruses have been sought for the cause of diseases in the recent past and the diseases – Legionnaire's and Lyme disease come to mind – were later found to be caused by bacteria. It is interesting to remember that Willy Burgdorfer, who identified the spirochete which causes Lyme disease, was in part alerted to the theory that it might be caused by a bacterium because penicillin was successful in relieving the symptoms of the disease.

It is possible that AIDS is caused by an infectious organism in a susceptible host and that the organism is a bacterium. This would explain the success of Stephen Caiazza and others in treating AIDS patients with antibiotics which are effective against bacteria. It would have to be an extremely small bacterium, less than .22 microns wide (that is, as small as a virus) because it would have to be able to pass through the extremely fine filter which is used to strain Factor VIII. Such bacteria certainly exist. It is possible, but the implications are so horrible it does not bear thinking about until there is further information. If a bacterial disease was misdiagnosed as a viral disease and all those people died because appropriate antibiotics were not used sufficiently aggressively, it would be the biggest disaster in medical history.

Seven

Origins

THE QUESTION OF where AIDS came from might be considered of academic interest only. Particularly from the point of view of the patient, the origin of the micro-organism responsible must be about as important as wondering how a fire started when one is standing in a burning building.

From the point of view of whether HIV causes AIDS, however, the issue is much more important. If it could be proved conclusively that AIDS existed widely at a time and place where there was no HIV infection, the theory would have to be re-evaluated. On the other hand, the theory is given tremendous support if the disease can be tracked via HIV infection to its source. This is why such great attention has been paid by HIV supporters to slave routes, African green monkeys and Portuguese sailors. He who controls the past controls the future. The history of AIDS, or the history of HIV, must hold the evidence as to whether this infection causes the disease.

Many theories of its origin are fanciful. All the leading ones are mentioned here.

From the skies

The most challenging theory of the origin of AIDS – ignoring the blatantly celestial – is that it is an epidemic sparked off by biological matter which exists in the upper atmosphere and is pulled to ground level by the patterns of global atmospheric circulation.

This proposal, by Sir Fred Hoyle and Chandra Wickramasinghe, follows these scientists' work on an origin in space for each new strain of influenza. They suggest that viral particles in the upper atmosphere are periodically augmented by comets carrying additional particles.

With this vast biological cloud effectively raining on the human race, it is inevitable that some viruses will 'take' and infect populations. Having worked out this model for the seasonal epidemics of influenza, it was relatively easy for Hoyle and Wickramasinghe to apply it to AIDS. Its sole advantage over other theories is that it explains the sporadic spread of the epidemic without having to refer to an individual carrier who initiated the epidemic – the quest for this 'Typhoid Mary' characterised the early days of AIDS epidemiology.

Fred Hoyle is a first-class scientist who has made fundamental contributions to astrophysics and cosmology, so it is sad to see his theories derided without examination by doctors who believe far stranger things about AIDS.

Under this theory, AIDS could be created by a virus which combined into a lethal form with other biological matter and with human tissue. HIV is not an essential element of it.

Conspiracies

The conspiracy theories of how AIDS began offer entertainment without enlightenment. The most frequently heard is that AIDS was the product of research into biological warfare which went disastrously wrong. This theory says that scientists at the US Defense Department's chemical and biological warfare research establishment at Fort Detrick, Maryland, experimented with genetically altered animal viruses in humans. A sheep virus called maedi-visna has been suggested as the starting point and in one particularly ghoulish variant it is said the 'guinea pigs' were people who were brain-dead but were kept 'alive' on life-support machines to observe the effect of the virus on human tissue.

The existence of research into biological warfare is not a secret. Defense Department testimony to a Washington appropriations committee in 1969 said: 'Within the next five or ten years, it would probably be possible to make a new infective micro-organism which could differ in certain respects from any known disease-causing organisms.

'Most important of these is that it might be refractory to the immunological and therapeutic properties upon which we depend to maintain our relative freedom from infectious disease.'

A report in the left-wing Californian paper *People's World* that the US Navy experimented with biological weapons aimed at black people never received substantiation.

Dr John Seale, a venereologist, feels the 'man-made virus' theory of the cause of AIDS is viable, though he does not believe a military aspect to the story is essential – it could have happened in an appropriately equipped biological sciences laboratory. He says:

> First and foremost, the means of transmission of AIDS are highly suggestive of a man-made virus. They are those which would be expected if a lethal animal retrovirus which causes persistent viraemia, such as maedi-visna, equine infectious anaemia, or simian AIDS virus, had been passaged *in vitro* [in the test tube] through human tissue culture, and then passaged *in vivo* [in the body] through humans used as guinea pigs. Visna virus was grown in cell culture of human astrocytes in the early nineteen-seventies and, according to eminent Soviet virologists, equine infectious anaemia virus can infect humans.

This theory can be examined in relation to the facts. Equine infectious anaemia virus causes anaemia (a low red blood count) in horses. Maedi-visna virus causes breathlessness and a brain infection in sheep. Both are of a family of viruses called lentiviruses. They are slow-acting animal viruses – they take an extended period to cause the diseases with which they are associated. It has been suggested that HIV is itself a lentivirus, so evidence supporting this theory would support HIV as the cause of AIDS. Or it could be that HIV was created in a lab but is still a harmless passenger virus. A virus has to come from somewhere, after all, whether or not it is pathogenic.

The conspiracy theory suggests that US researchers, perhaps with their Defense Department sponsors, released their biological bomb in Central Africa to see the result on human society. Another variant is that it 'escaped' from the laboratory or that it was tested on prisoners who volunteered for participation in medical experiments in order to increase their chances before the parole board. When the prisoners were released, perhaps into precisely the world of drug addiction where AIDS flourishes, they released the virus too.

Supporting evidence for the conspiracy theory came from a report that a CIA officer handed a Cuban émigré a canister containing biological material telling him to return to Cuba secretly and release it. The CIA almost certainly did cause epidemics in Cuba, including the dengue fever outbreak, and this story may be confusing those events with AIDS, the new flavour of the month for conspiracy theorists. It has a strong whiff of Soviet misinformation about it – 'I am from the CIA. Take this canister and poison Cuba with it and don't talk to any journalists about this.'

In some versions of this 'CIA subversion' conspiracy theory the virus introduced into Cuba was African swine fever virus (which will be dealt with later) and ASFV certainly did break out in Cuba in 1971. The Cubans then took the virus to Africa where they were fighting in Angola.

The argument against all this is that Cuba has a very low level of AIDS – six cases were recorded up to the middle of October 1987. The conspiracy theorists respond (there is always a response from con- spiracy theorists) that the animal virus was incubated in people and turned into a killer virus by a means which kept it isolated from the rest of the Cuban population. This centres on the Mariella boat lift when homosexuals, prostitutes, criminals and other 'undesirables' were thrown out of Cuba in 1980. Prior to this they had been held in prisons in Cuba. The theory is that the homosexuals spent their time in prison having sex with each other. A potentially harmless virus was incubated from person to person in this restricted community, mutating as it went, until a killer virus was produced. When the prisoners arrived in Florida, the homosexuals in particular found a welcome in the US gay community where they were settled in cities all over the country. The Sisters of Perpetual Indulgence, for example, the San Francisco performance artists who dress as nuns, did considerable work in ensuring that the refugees were housed in California.

Thus the killer virus spread throughout the community. While this theory superficially fits with the facts – the 'infected' homosexuals arrived at nearly the same time as the epidemic – the timing is not quite right, AIDS preceded the boat lift. Moreover, the Centers for Disease Control did meticulous epidemiological work in the early years of the epidemic; they would have noticed if there had been a preponderance of Cubans or of people with sexual contact with Cubans in the early samples.

Conspiracy theories suggesting that AIDS was a Soviet creation have never got off the ground. The fact that people gossiping in the US would rather blame their own side than their ostensible enemy says a great deal for the esteem in which Americans hold their political establishment.

Most of the conspiracy theories would not threaten HIV as the most favoured option for the cause of AIDS. Only the 'conspiracy arm' of the African swine fever virus theory does. The theory, however, can be seen on its own merits as the result of serious lab work and meticulous reasoning. It does not have to be seen – and dismissed – as a conspiracy theory.

African swine fever virus

The theory that a variant of African swine fever virus causes AIDS is of interest not so much because it is likely to be correct as for the light it sheds on the behaviour of the AIDS establishment when someone who wasn't invited started to play the game.

Jane Teas is a scientist who in 1983 was working at the Harvard School of Public Health in Boston. She had travelled considerably and was not constrained by any excessive bias towards one culture or one theory of disease.

She noticed a close parallel between the first cases of AIDS in Haiti and the appearance of African swine fever at the end of the nineteen-seventies.

African swine fever causes fever in infected pigs, followed by loss of appetite; increased amounts of gamma globulin in the blood, and enlargement of the lymphatic system. This last symptom could be compared to the swelling of the lymph nodes in patients with AIDS and other illnesses.

African swine fever infects lymphocytes and macrophages, which are key features of the immune system. Infected pigs suffer opportunistic infections because of their weakened immune systems and die when the infection is first introduced at a rate of almost one hundred per cent. The fatality rate then falls to only three per cent.

The virus is passed in bites from infected ticks to pigs; and from pigs to pigs by sex and orally through infected faeces, urine or meat.

People in Haiti often live in close proximity to domestic animals, including pigs. The pig is very close to humans in terms of its physiology, though this particular animal virus had not been known to infect humans before.

Jane Teas suggested in a letter to the *Lancet* in April 1983 that the Haitians got the virus from the pigs and spread it to 'sex tourists' who came from the US to enjoy Haitian night life.

'Perhaps an infected pig was killed and eaten either as uncooked or undercooked meat. One of the people eating the meat who was both immunocompromised and homosexual would be the pivotal point, allowing for the disease to spread to the vacationing "gay" tourists in Haiti.'

The geographical distribution of reported AIDS cases and ASFV outbreaks made this theory look promising. Anecdotal information from Haiti was supportive: Haitian AIDS patients who knew the pig disease well recognised that they had the same thing. But because of this coincidence, Haitian doctors had already tested the theory. Before Jane Teas thought about it, six Haitian doctors and a representative of the US Department of Agriculture had tested the blood of eight Haitian AIDS patients and four healthy controls to see if there were antibodies against ASFV. There were not.

One person who was stimulated by Jane Teas's work was John Beldekas, a chunky, forceful scientist at the Microbiology Department of Boston University's School of Medicine. He had been working with Foscarnet, a Swedish drug which was showing interesting lab results in work on tissue from AIDS patients. He found that adding Foscarnet to the malfunctioning white blood cells of AIDS patients made them return to normal. In searching the literature on Foscarnet he found the drug was effective against African swine fever in pigs. It was actually rarely used because it was cheaper to slaughter infected pigs than treat them but the drug was effective nevertheless.

John Beldekas called Jane Teas and they teamed up to research the theory further. John Beldekas started experiments in which he took samples from AIDS patients and mixed them with blood from pigs, finding the reaction in the pig blood was similar to its reaction when infected with ASFV. There were therefore some similarities between AIDS and the disease caused by ASFV. He then tested the pig blood which had been infected with tissue from AIDS patients and found it positive for antibodies specific to African swine fever virus.

The situation now began to get difficult. Jane Teas and John Beldekas were raising the question of whether there was African swine fever virus in pigs in the US. The US Department of Agriculture denied it despite the evidence from slaughterhouse surveys that pigs in New York, New Jersey and Texas had come into contact with the virus.

John Beldekas received two visits from US Department of Agriculture employees, one to take samples and inspect his findings and the next to discuss with him the importance of his work to the pork industry.

The reason the Department of Agriculture had to be involved was that they were the only people permitted to hold samples of ASFV from which reagents could be made to test for the presence of the virus. Reagents are testing substances – they always give the same chemical reaction when in contact with the matter to be analysed, in this case the virus.

African swine fever is a disease the Department of Agriculture was always keen to see kept out of the US, so samples of the virus were kept under tight security at the Exotic Animal Disease Research Facility at Plum Island, New York.

Jane Teas said:

When I first began my requests to the USDA and to Centers for Disease Control, I was told bluntly that no one in the United States would be willing to do such tests and that if I wanted any co-operation, I would have to go outside of this country. I have written letters to the Ministries of Health in Australia, the Cameroon and South Africa. I have visited the Food and Agriculture Organisation in Rome, to speak with the head of their animal testing service. In addition, I have visited the Ministry of Health in Italy, Spain and the Animal Research Institute in England and the Ministry of Health in Uganda.

Jane Teas's response from these organisations was disappointing, often after a promising start, which gave rise to allegations of a conspiracy against the African swine fever virus theory. The belief was that researchers in other countries had been agreeable to working with Jane Teas until US government officials called to frighten them off.

I have examined the events as carefully as I could for evidence of undue pressure but have not been able to substantiate the claims of a conspiracy as such. The failure to have work done in other countries can be explained by the authorities in those countries simply thinking that if the theory were that strong, why didn't research proceed in the US? Moreover, an individual woman scientist without the backing of a large research organisation would suffer a considerable degree of bias against her.

One of the people cited as having evidence of the conspiracy, William Hess, is the world expert on African swine fever. He works at Plum Island and he was cited at one time as having been present at a meeting in which the means to sabotage Teas and Beldekas' work had been discussed. When I asked him about this he said:

There wasn't a meeting, it was just someone at my level saying the work shouldn't go on. I was making statements that the work should be done. It warranted further research and I don't think they were able to do it with the facilities they had. They should have gone after the virus, until you have isolated the virus all you've got is a relationship. The serological [blood] studies are inadequate.

John Beldekas was working on the AIDS project at Boston University and when he went off on the swine connection there were people who thought he was going astray. There was enough evidence that it should have been looked at early on.

Teas and Beldekas enjoyed the support of the aggressive *New York Native*, the only lay publication, at least on the East Coast, which followed the AIDS story with any thoroughness. Their pressure, and as a knock-on effect that of other papers which ran the story after the *Native*, persuaded Plum Island to give John Beldekas a supply of African swine fever virus reagents with which to test patients.

He tested for the presence of the virus, a more appropriate test than that for antibodies which the human system produces to protect itself from the virus. Previous studies, including the Haitian study had looked for antibody and not for the virus. Tests were positive for nine out of twenty-one patients. One of sixteen controls was positive. On a note of caution he wrote in the *Lancet*: 'Since African swine fever virus infects only an estimated one per cent of macrophages at any one time, large sample sizes, special target assay systems, and several tests may be required to show an effect if ASFV and AIDS are really related.'

Jane Teas now became interested in an outbreak of AIDS in a particularly impoverished part of Florida called Belle Glade. There were forty-nine cases in a town of 15,000 people. Two enthusiastic researchers were attempting to interest the AIDS establishment in Belle Glade because it was so unusual – nineteen of the victims had no apparent risk factors.

These two doctors, Caroline MacLeod and Mark Whiteside, insisted that the prevalence of AIDS in Belle Glade meant environmental factors had to have something to do with the disease.

MacLeod said: 'It makes me so angry when they try to put everything in categories and make it simple. It is going to be like consumption in the eighteen-hundreds which was all different kinds of pneumonia – TB was just one of them. There were bacterial infections, viral infections, fungal infections. It is ultimately going to be all sorts of different diseases working together, different patterns, different presentations.'

The AIDS establishment viewed this kind of remark with disdain. AIDS was going to be caused by one microbe, they would isolate it, develop a vaccine, produce some drugs and there would be no more problem. The thought that environmental conditions might have anything to do with AIDS was anathema.

John Beldekas tested ten Belle Glade pigs and found one positive for African swine fever virus. The Department of Agriculture first confirmed the results then re-ran the tests and was able to proclaim it was 'satisfied that African swine fever does not exist in Belle Glade'.

These events had reached the mainstream press and a reporter for the *New York Times* wrote a story which had severe implications for John Beldekas's career. The reporter asked John if it were possible that his test result was a false positive: that the test had shown positive for African swine fever virus which was not in fact there. He replied that of course it was possible. The reporter wrote: 'Presumably, Mr Beldekas' diagnosis was a false positive; he now acknowledges that he may have confused a standard positive test serum with his sample.' John Beldekas insists that he only remarked in response to a direct question that an event was possible, he did not present it as a realistic history.

Unfortunately when a subject is in print, it assumes a status often quite out of proportion to its true importance. John Beldekas's senior colleagues did not like to see him admitting in public that his research could have been sloppy. He had been trying their patience with his African swine fever story anyway. He did not remain in his job.

Jane Teas continued looking at Belle Glade. Having found no

correlation between pigs and AIDS cases – most of the victims had not come into contact with pigs, infected or otherwise – there had to be some other carrier for the virus if the African swine fever virus theory was going to stand up. The only other known vector for the virus was ticks. So Jane Teas looked for ticks on the pigs – perhaps the ticks had bitten the pigs then the people. She was unable to find ticks there or in the chickens or in the many rats around Belle Glade.

She found some ticks in turtle burrows sixty miles from Belle Glade but was unable to find a lab willing to test them for infected blood. The story was getting remote by now, and anyway insect vectors for AIDS had been discounted a long time before. Insects don't bite only the sexually active, AIDS does.

There were other trickles of news like the New York State Department of Health testing the blood in its blood bank and finding that 4.5 per cent of it contained antibodies to African swine fever virus. The Centers for Disease Control tested the sera of AIDS patients which they had stored and found some positives for African swine fever virus but declared they must have been mistaken. This information came out only as a result of two congressional inquiries. Jane Teas said: 'I do not doubt their right to their opinion, but I strongly object to their decision not to publish their information, along with their methodology and results. I want more from my government than science behind closed doors.'

The theory was struggling along; there wasn't sufficient new fact to support it. If African swine fever was a significant factor in AIDS, there ought to be a good deal more of it about. Antibodies to HIV were claimed to be present in up to ninety per cent of patients; African swine fever virus had only ever managed just under 50 per cent in a small cohort of patients. Of course, if people were not looking for the virus, they wouldn't find it; but it seemed clear that some researchers, such as the CDC, had looked, albeit surreptitiously. It is as well to remember what the theory was aiming at. John Beldekas told the Press Association: 'I don't think we're trying to say that (HIV) is out and ASFV is in. What we're saying is that AIDS is complicated. It can't be explained solely by (HIV). There's another cog in the wheel.'

There was no funding for further work. Jane Teas was out of work for a year. Beldekas found another job but was warned to keep his private interest in African swine fever virus to himself – even though he was in charge of a department which was testing the blood of AIDS patients and healthy people. Teas finally felt she had paid enough in personal terms for her work on that theory.

Jane Teas and John Beldekas demonstrated that African swine fever can infect humans, which is no small achievement. This cannot be taken as conclusive because the virus has not been isolated from human blood, but, nevertheless, a little nugget of fact has been placed in the canon of science.

The real problem for this theory and the reason why it was never taken seriously, was that the big money was already on a retrovirus. From 1982, before Jane conceived the theory, decisions had been made which made it inevitable that a retrovirus like HIV would be found in AIDS patients. It was all the laboratories were looking for. Jane Teas and John Beldekas had done the scientific equivalent of walking into a casino where punters were betting tens of thousands of dollars on every turn of the wheel and trying to change the rules of the game while putting down a stake of a week's wages.

As John Beldekas said:

There's a tremendous resistance here to pursue unorthodox scientific ideas. Even though we had good solid proof. It was just excluded without any reason. They just thought it was a bad idea. They accused Dr Teas of having wrong thinking, they accused me of being a lunatic fringe scientist in addition to being an out of the closet homosexual. There was a political and a scientific agenda to prevent this going further.

They don't harm you, they just prevent you from doing further research. I was basically asked to leave Boston University School of Medicine because certain individuals thought it was embarrassing that my work was done there.

It wasn't the pork industry either. We never mentioned the pork industry. The farmers weren't upset because we weren't talking about pork causing AIDS, we were talking about an animal virus but, if you're trying to discredit somebody, you use all different types of means. The idea that there was a threat to the pork industry was just another way of putting pressure on us.

AIDS and the vaccination programme

The theory that AIDS was spread by the re-use of needles in the vaccination programmes operated in the Third World at least relies on clinical observation in a real patient.

Don was a nineteen-year-old black man from the mid-southwestern US. He had always been fit, taking part in high school competitive athletics with ease. Don was an ordinary, street-wise young man, he wasn't an angel, but he didn't do anything crazy. He had been having sex with girls since he was fourteen, increasingly frequently in more recent years, sometimes with prostitutes. He had never injected drugs. There was no reason why he shouldn't be allowed to join the army, which he did in April 1984, medical examination finding him a perfect physical specimen.

Though smallpox has been eradicated in the world, in part due to a major World Health Organization drive in the nineteen-seventies, 'the vaccine continues to be given to certain military populations worldwide because of strategic defensive military and antiterrorist considerations,' the *New England Journal of Medicine* remarked. This means an army could still fight even if the other side released the droplet-borne smallpox virus over their camp. Likewise, if a terrorist organisation laid hands on a canister of smallpox and threatened to release it, there would be a vaccinated population which could deal with the crisis.

Don duly received vaccinations against adenoviruses 4 and 7, measles, rubella, a form of influenza, polio, a form of meningitis, tetanus, diphtheria and smallpox. Don had been born too late to have received 'primary vaccination' against smallpox at school, the programme had already been discontinued by the time he was ready to have the shot. He therefore had to have the smallpox vaccine for the first time as an adult – clearly recognised as a more dangerous procedure than vaccination for children.

Don was unaffected by the vaccinations. He participated fully in basic training for the next two and a half weeks; then he developed a temperature, blinding headaches, neck stiffness. At night his sheets were soaked in sweat. On 30 May he was transferred to Walter Reed Army Medical Center.

He had meningitis (inflammation of the outer tissues of the brain); lymphadenopathy measured by his swollen lymph glands; oral thrush and low levels of T helper cells.

Four weeks after vaccination, while receiving treatment for his meningitis, a huge ulcer, three by four centimetres across, developed on the vaccination site. Over the next two or three days, pustules came up all over his buttocks and legs, rapidly becoming ulcerated. He was developing the disease the vaccine had been aimed to prevent.

He was given treatment for the 'vaccinia' and they were healed by mid-August. Over the next three months the oral thrush resolved and the T helper cells went up. Don was feeling better.

Then his helper T cell count started to go down again, the thrush returned and he became increasingly confused, forgetful, he no longer seemed to have control over his body. His brain was being destroyed.

He lived on, in increasing misery, until December 1985.

The doctors reporting on the case felt that HIV, which their patient had, was accelerated from its dormant state by the vaccines. Damage from vaccines is a common phenomenon, usually overlooked by public health authorities who accept that the individual must suffer for the general good, though the individual is never asked to comment on this state of affairs. As the doctors in this case noted, referring to the Advisory Committee on Immunization Practices: 'Although the Committee acknowledges the concern about the potential role of immunisation-induced deterioration, it believes that the potential benefits of immunisation of infected children by means of killed vaccines outweigh this theoretical adverse event.'

The authors did, however, raise a question over the widespread use of vaccination in Africa. This was taken up by others who indicated it could give an indication of the spread of AIDS. As Pearce Wright, science editor of the London *Times* wrote: 'It would account for the position of each of the seven Central African states which top the league table of most-affected countries; why Brazil became the most afflicted Latin American country; and how Haiti became the route for the spread of AIDS to the US.

'It also provides an explanation of how the infection was spread more evenly between males and females in Africa than in the West and why there is less sign of infection among five to eleven year olds in Central Africa.' The vaccination programme was stopped, having been judged a success, just as the eleven-year-olds of 1987 were reaching an age when vaccination would be possible.

Needles were used forty to sixty times, being waved across a flame between injections to sterilise them.

The World Health Organization reacted with horror at this proposition that their good intentions had so backfired. There were immediate and aggressive denials, claiming the low incidence of AIDS in Asia was evidence against transmission by inoculation. It was no such thing, of course. If there wasn't a great deal of the agent which causes AIDS in Asia in the first place, there wasn't a great deal to be amplified. If there was a lot in Africa, there were many more chances of it being passed on.

The WHO also unconvincingly remarked that people are receiving a small number of injections during inoculation and that the needles are small and can carry only a tiny amount of contaminated blood. People supporting the HIV hypothesis have always claimed only one dose is needed and the size of the needle should hardly be an issue – drug addicts do not use gigantic needles and they pass on AIDS.

The Paris-based National Association for Freedom from Vaccination understandably seized on this subject. Their director Simone Delarue wrote: 'We can recall in the nineteen-sixties when antipolio vaccines were heavily contaminated with a monkey virus called SV 40. In 1980 Krieg and his collaborators recovered fragments of SV 40 from a number of human cerebral tumours. This result went to confirm research by Heinonen of 1973 when the rate of cerebral cancer among the children of 50,000 women studied between 1959 and 1965, thirty-six per cent of whom had been vaccinated against polio during pregnancy, was thirteen times the rate for children whose mothers had not been vaccinated.'

The problem with this sort of theory is that it can never be 'proved', further information can be drafted in to support it but chasing these theories leads to more and more information which is less and less conclusive.

A far higher risk in Africa were the 'inoculators' who sold injections in bars and market places. A belief in the potency of injections has led to a massive quack industry in Africa where vitamins and antibiotics are injected for a small payment as a cure for minor ailments, as a tonic and for the usual condition for which bogus medicine is prescribed: impotence.

Disposable syringes have added to the problem in that they are not disposed of after use in Africa but are re-used. On 1 April 1987 Unicef banned the supply of disposable syringes to countries which couldn't prove they threw them away after one use, but in a continent with a vast private market in medicines and medical implements, it seems unlikely that official actions will have any great effect.

The vaccination-AIDS theory has been used to shore up HIV against one of the most telling criticisms of it: that though most AIDS patients have at one time been infected by HIV, it is far too weak a virus to cause the damage characteristic of AIDS.

To quote *The Times* again: 'Other doctors who accept the connection between the anti-smallpox campaign and the AIDS epidemic now see answers to questions which had baffled them. How, for instance, the AIDS organism, previously regarded by scientists as "weak, slow and vulnerable", began to behave like a type capable of creating a plague.'

The idea is that vaccination turned a minor illness of the nineteen-seventies into the epidemic of the nineteen-eighties. It is compatible with other theories of AIDS development but it does not explain where the original infection came from, and whether or not that infection is HIV.

African monkeys

The theory of the origin of AIDS which has enjoyed the most success is that it is a crossover from an African green monkey which once bit a person in Central Africa who then developed a lethal human form of a harmless monkey virus.

The wide circulation of this theory owes a great deal to the fact that it was proposed by Myron (Max) Essex, a close colleague of the leading US AIDS researcher Robert Gallo.

In November 1985 Max Essex and co-workers published information about a virus they had found in healthy wild-caught African green monkeys. It was structurally similar to HIV (though it was referred to as HTLV-III at that time) and it was therefore called STLV-III, the S standing for 'simian' as the H stood for 'human'.

The problem was that it didn't cause AIDS in the monkey, or any disease, it seemed. Despite its similarity to the virus said to be causing the present epidemic, STLV-III was a harmless passenger virus. This might have made the researchers think twice about whether HIV was a similarly harmless virus, but if it did there is no mention of this in their paper. They ploughed on: 'The study of STLV-III in African green monkeys may . . . lead to the development of a model system for the study and prevention of AIDS.'

This was massaging one of the sore points about the theory that HIV causes AIDS: there is no animal model for it. No laboratory animal has ever been given HIV and gone on to develop AIDS. Only people get it. Perhaps experiments with monkeys on a morphologically similar virus to HIV might be acceptable.

The situation then began to get complicated. France's leading AIDS researcher Luc Montagnier described another strain of HIV in two AIDS patients from West Africa. If the original HIV came from a bite from the African green monkey, where did these two get their virus from?

Joe Sonnabend, a founder of the AIDS Medical Foundation in New York and champion of the view that AIDS is not caused by a single factor, was derisive:

> It's a very simplistic interpretation to think that the origin of HIV was in a monkey which at some momentous occasion bit somebody and caused a virus epidemic.
>
> It's particularly untenable at the moment because we have a virus called HIV2 and it has a sixty per cent difference from HIV1. We're not speaking of small strain differences, these are different viruses. These two different viruses are said to cause a similar disease. Well, that's not unknown, we do have hepatitis and some other clinical conditions that can be produced by different viruses but end up causing the same disease.
>
> However, if HIV1 came from a simian virus then HIV2 presumably came from a simian virus, now we need two monkey bites. Not only do we need two monkey bites, but they have to have

occurred in the same time frame. That's absurd. The scenario of the monkey bite as producing this epidemic is just a fantasy.

The second possible point of crossover was mentioned in a letter to the *Lancet*. It refers to an account written by anthropologist Anicet Kashamura about the sexual habits of the people of the Great Lakes region of Central Africa: 'To stimulate a man or a woman and induce them to intense sexual activity, monkey blood or she monkey blood was inoculated into the thighs, pubic area and back.'

Abraham Karpas, a prominent British AIDS researcher, feels this is a helpful contribution to the debate which explains how there were two strains of HIV. He wrote: 'The difference between HIV1 (of Central African origin) and HIV2 (of West African origin) could be explained in terms of the tribes in Central Africa using the blood of a different species of monkey for injection.' Karpas also notes with some disdain the practice of 'monkey glands' being injected into affluent Europeans. He suggests that, because the rejuvenation therapy is unlikely to have had any effect, 'the ageing patients were in no position to spread any new virus to mankind.'

There is no evidence of how widespread the practice of inoculating with monkey blood to increase virility was in Africa. Indeed, with the exception of Kashamura's paper, I know of no evidence that it ever happened. As one commentator put it: 'People are notoriously good at making up weird habits to please or fool inquisitive scientists. And the monkey blood method may be far from typical: it may simply be an individual's perversion that the researcher stumbled across.'

There are frequent anecdotal references, generally verbal and accompanied by sniggers, that sex between monkeys and men may have been responsible for the species crossover. Sex between men and monkeys in Africa is not commonly reported. I have not heard it referred to outside the reference in connection with AIDS. Doubtless bestiality occurs in Africa as it does in England, but the absence of evidence for it (compare Arabia, where the anecdotal evidence is vast) suggests it is so rare as to be discounted.

Another reason makes this method of communication of a virus unlikely. Jane Teas, whose PhD research was in primatology, explained it to me. 'Do you know how big they are?' she asked, indicating with her hand the height of, say, a squatting six-year-old child, 'and they are mean critters. No one in their right mind would try to hump an African green monkey.'

A more promising suggestion is a crossover from monkeys used for tissue culture research and for the preparation of vaccines which were then, of course, injected into the bloodstream of millions. Two Italian researchers wrote in *Nature*:

In the nineteen-fifties, the introduction of tissue cultures in research into human enteroviruses, and in studies of the preparation and control of polio vaccines, caused a massive request for monkeys, and many primate stabularies were created where different species of monkeys often lived together. African green monkey has been one of the monkeys used most for kidney cultures for enterovirus studies.

This caused an unprecedented human manipulation of African green monkeys by Africans involved in the capture and maintenance of these monkeys and stabulary and laboratory personnel of western countries. All this might have vastly increased the odds of an accidental passage of (the simian virus) from African green monkeys to other monkeys and to humans.

Support for this theory of the origin of AIDS came from the British National Anti-Vivisection Society, which produced a report in 1987 giving detailed accounts of laboratory manipulation of viruses and the experimental infection of monkeys. *Biohazard – The Silent Threat from Biomedical Research and the Creation of AIDS* gives an impressive amount of circumstantial information about 'AIDS-like' illnesses in laboratory strains of monkeys going back to 1969. The report did not receive the attention it merited, presumably because it came from a source which was so obviously inimical to a great deal of laboratory practice. It obviously had a case to make, but since every published theory is pushing a particular case, the concept of an 'unbiased' theory is a contradiction in terms.

The alternative view to all this is that, just as HIV is a harmless passenger virus which does not cause AIDS, a retrovirus has been isolated from monkeys which also does not cause AIDS. Given time, retroviruses could be isolated from many other species, and they wouldn't cause AIDS either.

The blood dealers

A corollary to the African origin of AIDS theory is the view that it was spread into the West by the activities of international plasma dealers. They would buy blood products from the poor, complete with their crop of blood-borne infections including AIDS, and would sell them to the rich.

The basis for this trade is plasmapheresis. This is a fast and efficient means of taking white cells from a blood donor while leaving the red cells, which take longer for the body to replace naturally. In a Third World country a donor will be paid to lie down while a quantity of blood is taken from his arm. The plasmapheresis machine which takes the blood then centrifuges it to separate white from red blood cells and returns the red cells to the donor. The white cells are then frozen in a bag and sent to a country rich enough to afford a fractionating plant that will separate the plasma into its component parts which can then be used for treatment: Factor VIII, Factor IX, gamma globulin and so on.

Peter Jones of the Newcastle Haemophilia Centre in England notes that the plasmapheresis centres supplying Western companies in the nineteen-seventies 'were situated in exactly the areas now known to be endemic for Kaposi's sarcoma and other AIDS-related diseases'. One of the main centres for plasmapheresis was Kinshasa, the capital of Zaire which has sometimes been seen to be at the centre of AIDS in Africa. Others were in Ghana, the Congo, the Ivory Coast and Senegal. In Latin America there were centres in Nicaragua, Belize and Haiti.

'Given the long incubation period for AIDS,' Jones continued, 'these facts suggest that the disease was introduced into the United States not by sexual transmission but via plasma obtained in endemic areas. The exposure of a population with no natural resistance and with a proclivity to promiscuity resulted in its spread.'

This theory enjoyed great goodwill in that people were positive about its possibility and the blood brokers were not popular. But attempts to give it more validity failed utterly. After months of research no fragment of evidence further than that circumstantial material which Peter Jones reports was forthcoming.

There are a number of arguments against this theory, of which the general lack of evidence to support it is only one. It relies on an African origin of AIDS and it seems increasingly clear as we near the end of the eighties that AIDS appeared in Africa and America at roughly the same time. If AIDS first came in through plasma, moreover, the first hit would have been haemophiliacs, not heroin addicts and homosexuals. It has been suggested that this might have been the case but haemophiliacs built up a resistance to the AIDS agent – they were getting small amounts of contaminated material over a long period rather than one large inoculation which intravenous drug users or highly promiscuous homosexuals get; they therefore took longer to die though they had been infected earlier.

Another suggestion was that a homosexual haemophiliac got the AIDS agent in imported plasma and had spread it into the homosexual community by promiscuous sex before he himself died, though his death was not classified as an AIDS death because no epidemic had been recognised at that time and haemophiliacs anyway have a high mortality rate.

The problem here is that the suggestion is getting further and further away from verifiable facts in order to substantiate a theory which is itself based on a number of assumptions.

I was most convinced of the watery nature of this story when I spoke to Dennis Donahue, who had been responsible for the regulation of blood products for the Food and Drug Administration of the USA.

He said, 'There have been stories about contaminated plasma going back to the mid-seventies. Since then there have been substantial changes in regulations which mean if the stories were ever true, they are not any longer.'

Did AIDS arrive from abroad in contaminated plasma? I would think it unlikely. There was a lot of perception that plasma came from Central America. A substantial proportion was from a facility located in Nicaragua. It was not derived from the black population of the Caribbean who had contact with Africans or from Africans themselves.

In other words, what plasma there was from abroad came from areas where AIDS was not and is not endemic.

Moreover, it is known that heavily infected populations – heroin users and homosexuals – were donating plasma in the late seventies and early eighties. The heroin users were doing it for money – commercial plasmapheresis units all over New York's notorious Lower East Side, for example, were paying around ten dollars a unit for plasma. The payment for plasma was flexible throughout the US: when supplies were low, blood dealers would increase the payment to encourage more indigent people to step up and donate.

The homosexuals donated from goodwill – as part of the campaign against hepatitis B.

Dennis Donahue takes a point of view which is often stated as a scientific principle: if there is a simple and easily available explanation for a phenomenon, why look for a complicated one?

'We do not need to look abroad to find sources of transmission of AIDS,' he says.

Plasma was being collected from prisons and in the hearts of the major cities where AIDS was first recognised as an epidemic. It was also collected from cities which were used by the male homosexual population – that plasma was used in preparing gamma globulin for inoculation against hepatitis. For that reason, as soon as it was realised that AIDS was a problem, there was no more unsterilised plasma collected for that use as from December 1982.

Of course, the most cynical would say Donahue was just covering his back. He had been responsible for plasma and should have ensured its safety. But no one would accuse a person of negligence for being unaware of the transmissibility of AIDS in blood products in 1979 or

1980. Moreover, in accepting the routes which were instrumental in contaminating blood products, Donahue does acknowledge a means of transmission which he had some responsibility for.

The role of the blood dealers in the spread of AIDS remains an intriguing topic for speculation and it would please me greatly to see a trial by media of a guilty blood products company. I have not seen the evidence to prove even that a crime has been committed, however, and am in no position to name the guilty man.

Lifestyle

Theories about the origin of AIDS need to take account of people like Robert R. He died of AIDS in 1969 in St Louis, Missouri. Robert, sixteen, was admitted to a clinic in 1968 with swollen lymph nodes. He suffered weight loss and fatigue and a severe infection with Chlamydia. He had only one visible lesion of Kaposi's sarcoma, on his thigh, but when he died of pneumonia the autopsy showed other lesions throughout the soft tissues of his body.

Robert was sexually active and it was noticed that he suffered lesions around the anus and chronic haemorrhoids, common among highly active homosexuals. It is suggested that he was a male prostitute.

Doctors were so puzzled by his death that they kept the tissue in the hope a diagnosis could be made in the future.

The diagnosis was made in October 1987. Robert R's blood did contain antibodies to HIV, which satisfies those who believe in the HIV hypothesis, though old blood is now notorious for giving false results to tests.

Robert R. had clearly experienced the life of drugs and sex which became associated with AIDS more than a decade later. At the time Robert R. was alive, there were already warning signs of the physical toll which the 'fast track' lifestyle was taking. Professor Gordon Stewart was an observer of these signs in the late 60s. Gordon Stewart had worked on the new range of penicillins and cephalosporins in the nineteen-fifties and was largely responsible for alerting the medical profession and the public to the dangers of pertussis (whooping cough) vaccine. In 1968–71 as Watkins Professor of Epidemiology at Tulane University in New Orleans he received a grant from the National Institute of Mental Health to study drug addiction in New Orleans and New York City.

His team there was studying behavioural rather than pathological aspects of drug addiction in addicts as compared to control subjects but an experienced clinician could not but note the range of infections the addicts had:

They were getting all sorts of opportunistic infections, probably passed on by needles – eighty-five to ninety per cent of them had evidence of hepatitis. They were often extremely emaciated, suffering from wasting diseases, various weird blood-borne infections with skin bacteria, Candida and Cryptococci, which would not ordinarily be regarded as pathogenic in their own right.

Many of them were blood donors – they would get paid for their blood and they didn't mind giving it. They didn't mind needles, some of them like needles.

We didn't find Kaposi's sarcoma and we didn't find Pneumocystis (carinii pneumonia) but, then, we weren't looking for it.

One way to test for Pneumocystis is by an open lung biopsy – an expensive surgical technique which would be unlikely to be lavished on the poor. The other method is bronchoscopy in which a tube is passed down the windpipe into the bronchial tubes where material is aspirated or a small piece of tissue is cut out and brought up for laboratory analysis.

Darrell Yates Rist, journalist and observer of New York life, said:

New York research into intravenous drug use shows no suspicious deaths before 1976 but that research was done on death certificates. Someone reports the death of a junkie, the body is taken away and put down as overdose. No one is going to do an open lung smear on that person to find out if they really died of pneumocystis. Injection is also a much more efficient method of passing on the infection. You get it straight into your bloodstream. Sexual transmission seems to be far more dose-related – reinfection seems to be a central point as well, you need more than one contact.

The intravenous drug users were in the lead and only later the gays picked it up. The first case of AIDS I know of in the US was in 1976 when the baby of an IV drug user died of pneumocystis in San Francisco.

The failure of American society to develop a comprehensive system of free medical care contributed to a large degree to the spread of AIDS in the early years. Many patients unable to afford medical care continued to suffer with their disease, almost certainly transmitting it to others, up to the point of their death.

It was the industrious and relatively affluent white homosexual community, with its income free from the demands of wives and children, which first paid to see doctors and visit hospitals with complaints which were, at that time, less than fatal.

The drug addicts and Haitians died unnoticed, as Dr Stephen Joseph, Health Commissioner of New York, confirmed in October 1987 when he added 2520 deaths among IV drug users, mainly blacks and Hispanics, to the official AIDS death list. They had been overlooked, or, 'not identified by surveillance'.

Fifty-three per cent of people with AIDS in New York City in 1987 were black or hispanic.

A typical early case of AIDS which preceded an understanding of the epidemic is described by Donald Louria of the New Jersey Medical School. He saw a thirty-year-old female drug addict and prostitute who had extreme difficulty in swallowing because of the Candida in her mouth and throat. She had suffered the usual weight loss and fever. She soon died from pneumonia. Dr Louria said: 'Although no autopsy was performed, we realised one year later that she had almost certainly suffered from AIDS and that the unexplained lethal pneumonia was probably due to Pneumocystis carinii.'

In New York the stench of poverty is evident as perhaps in no other Western city. In the US the desperate conditions of perhaps ten per cent of the entire population do not excite a great deal of comment. In a nation where the most popular explanation for poverty is personal failing, no one need care about their fellows falling by the wayside from Pneumocystis carinii pneumonia or any other cause.

In the Medicaid Center at 330 West 34th street, between 8th and 9th, thousands throng the hall every day where they wait for their number to be called to attend an interview where it will be decided if they qualify for limited free medical care. There are one and a half million New Yorkers on Medicaid at any one time. 'They must be too dumb to get health insurance,' said a woman at a dinner party where I happened to mention this.

Moreover, forty per cent of all applications to Medicaid in 1984 were refused, so we must be looking at well in excess of two million people who are so poor they either qualify for medical assistance or at least believe they do to such an extent that they are prepared to endure the humiliation of refusal.

New York is conspicuously wealthy with its furs and glittering towers and long, long limousines, but anyone who dares walk a few blocks up from the museum area on Central Park finds themselves in a place as desperate as a Third World shanty town – the rubbish piled in the street where a band of youths play ball, the despondent men who lean against graffiti-covered walls swapping shouts of greeting, the burned-out cars in the shadow of burned-out tenements where children play in scenes of Dickensian squalor.

As hospitals cannot refuse emergency treatment when it is needed, poor people present at the emergency department with conditions which are demonstrably not emergencies because it is a way of obtaining free medical treatment.

King's County Hospital in Brooklyn is the sort of building nightmares are set in. It is a huge, dark, bare institution of a place. In a crowded corridor leading to emergency, a man with gunshot wounds is being carried in a blood-soaked sheet. Workers are rushing and shouting and pushing through with samples and papers and trolleys. In an open space a long queue of Hispanic and black people snakes away from a wire mesh window where a young woman barks questions at them and hands out thermometers. Many more people are sitting, dejected and tired, in rows of wooden seats. Anyone wishing to film Dante's *Inferno* could set one hell scene here.

'There is a triage system,' I was told. 'If you are unconscious you get treatment immediately, if you are running a temperature it's a few hours, if you aren't obviously an emergency you just wait.'

'How long?'

'Five hours on a good day, maybe eight, maybe sixteen.'

A black man in a wheelchair saw my colleague put down a pie he had been eating. 'Are you going to finish that pie?'

'No, I've had enough.'

'Can I have it?'

The man wheeled off eating the remains of the pie. He hadn't been trying to elicit money by pretending to beg for food; he actually was hungry. In the richest nation in the world a sick man who couldn't afford health treatment was begging for food.

Several people, notably Joe Sonnabend, have characterised AIDS as a disease of poverty which has been present in the Third World for years when no one really cared what the people were dying of – there were so many deaths, who could bother to establish whether this one is Toxiplasma gondii or that one is caused by Mycobacterium avium intercellulare? This theory says AIDS was apparent in people living in Third World conditions in the US and became manifest in the homosexual community when they duplicated Third World conditions – lowered immunity, repeated re-infection with a variety of pathogens – in their bathhouses.

Eight

Africa

TO MOST PEOPLE, television is the main source of news and information about the world. As opposed to the cynicism which greets newspaper coverage, there is a touching faith in the truth value of television reports. This is particularly true of reports from abroad. Indeed, it seems the further away the country and the more remote the subject matter from life in their own backyard, the more credulous the TV audience.

Television journalists are believed to be expert in the field they cover. They are expected to display an assiduous regard for the truth and a selfless determination to obtain footage at whatever cost. In fact there are many more factors than journalistic resolve in the making of television programmes. The amount of time available, the comfort of the crew, the determination to get a hard story and interpersonal relationships all play a part. Most importantly, when dealing with foreign filming, there are the demands of the TV station itself. It costs a great deal of money to send a TV crew to another country. The pressure to bring back the story for which one was sent out, true or not, is irresistible.

Television journalists are rarely subjected to the fresh breeze of criticism which their cousins on newspapers enjoy so frequently. As TV journalists must bear at least some of the responsibility for the widespread misconceptions about AIDS in Africa, I have constructed a little fiction which explains some of the pressures on TV journalists working so far from home.

Interlude: The TV People

The director stared through the plate glass window at a vendor in the busy street outside the hotel. He needed an opening shot for his piece on

AIDS in Kenya. Perhaps the hands of the vendor, camera pulling out to show the range of goods and cigarettes he sold: 'In downtown Nairobi you can buy almost anything, you can buy a prostitute for a few pounds, but condoms are hard to come by and not many Africans use them,' he mused. No, too complicated, perhaps pulling back from some identifiably African object in a local shop to show a tourist looking in: 'Some Europeans will take back more than a souvenir from their holiday in Kenya.' That was more like it.

The director looked up as his colleagues joined him. The young woman whose title was production assistant went to the bar to buy lagers for them. The director was a man in his early forties. He had been in television all his life; he had started off in light entertainment as a sound trainee and had slowly moved up the promotion ladder of one of Britain's big television companies. He had been in current affairs for six years, mainly working on domestic stories for the regional news magazine. He had been to Africa once before, to take some film of the national settlement when Rhodesia became Zimbabwe. He had covered the Lancaster House conference in London the year before and they thought he deserved a trip abroad. This time he had been sent out because all other available directors were in other countries, also working on AIDS.

The researcher was a young man for whom it was the first trip abroad with the company. He had been doing public relations work and research for advertising agencies before he got into television. He got in by being chosen out of seventy serious applicants for the advertised post of researcher for a children's programme. Once in the company it was just a long slow push to get out of children's TV and into the more glamorous area of current affairs.

He knew a lot about AIDS in Africa. He had taken every appropriate cutting from the company's library of published articles. The researcher knew that fifty per cent of the people in the Turkana region of Kenya were positive for the AIDS virus; he knew that over eighty per cent of prostitutes in the poor area of Nairobi were infected. He knew that in late 1985 one large bank in Kinshasa had half its staff sick with AIDS. He knew that AIDS originated in Africa from an infected monkey bite and that the virus had then somehow transformed itself into a human virus. He knew Africa was the great centre of AIDS in the world, facing a plague of horrifying proportions. It was all very exciting.

The Kenyan interpreter was always referred to as 'Jimmy' because few of the foreign TV crews who visited could pronounce his African name. His cousin in the government had helped him get this job which basically consisted of babysitting TV crews – helping them to go where they wanted and discouraging them from offending local customs. They *all* wanted to film an AIDS victim's funeral. Funerals are big family matters in Kenya, he had to explain, they are very important, you cannot go with cameras. How did they conduct funerals in Europe, he wondered, did they have a lot of cameras? Still, there was a lot he did not understand. Why were they so interested in prostitutes all the time? Didn't they have prostitutes back home?

This was a good job. It carried a lot of weight with local people because they thought he told the TV crews what to do. It paid well and food was always provided by the crews. Just this month he had worked with the Swedish crew, the Germans and the ones from American TV who were always complaining. Now the British. All for the AIDS. Before the TV crews started coming, he had never seen anyone with the AIDS. In fact, if he didn't go round with the TV crews, he never would see anyone with the AIDS.

The production assistant actually knew quite a bit about Africa; she had visited several African countries for work and on holiday. Her brother-in-law was a Kenyan doctor and he had talked about AIDS with her and other family members.

Her job here was to draw up the timetable to make sure crew members were in the right place at the right time. The technical crew – the cameraman, his assistant, sound and lighting – would not, of course, attend an editorial meeting like this even though some of them had considerable African experience.

The production assistant would also take notes on the material which was being filmed, to assist in the editing process. It was she who had invented the title 'Aidsathon' to describe the current project, where AIDS in seven countries around the world was being covered in one programme. Each country would have a seven-minute film to describe the AIDS epidemic there, except America, which would get half an hour. Then there would be a studio discussion with the British health minister and some leading doctors. It would last two hours of prime time TV and would be put out on the network, just like the 'Telethon' programmes, hence Aidsathon.

She was probably the most intelligent person at the editorial meeting in the hotel bar but she was intellectually idle and tended to take options in life which minimised the need for complex thought. It was easier to be a production assistant and work out logistics which had attainable answers than to work on content which meant unpaid overtime and responsibility.

Though she knew more about Africa, and Kenya in particular, than her colleagues, no one asked her anything. The only thing you ever ask the PA, after all, is: 'Where are we going to stop for lunch?'

'OK, we've got three days,' said the director. 'Let's start early tomorrow and get the establishing shots of Nairobi done, have an early lunch and then get out to this AIDS clinic. We'd better shoot a victim or two and a caring doctor battling against the odds. Would you go in the morning', he said to the researcher, 'and make sure the victims know what's going to happen and we have their permission. I don't want people covering their faces or looking startled when we arrive. Just a nice hospital scene with a doctor comforting patients. If the doctor's got anything to say we'll mike him up for a few minutes of chat. And can you sort out some shortages shots, you know, empty cupboards where the linen and rubber gloves were stored, one syringe between ten patients, that sort of thing.'

'I'm not sure about the last bit,' said the researcher. 'This is Nairobi, not the jungle, they're not badly equipped here. We'll get the shortages stuff when we go out into the back of beyond.'

'Well, see what you can do,' said the director. 'Early start the next day and out to this typical village with dying people, what's it called?'

'Nakuru,' Jimmy said. It was a favourite of the TV people. It was possible to get there in a few hours, do some filming and be back at the hotel in Nairobi at night. Jimmy also had some sick people there for them. Someone had told him there were people there who were sick with the AIDS and he had gone to them and told them the TV people would pay to film them. He couldn't tell what had made the people sick but if it wasn't the AIDS it didn't matter, the TV people were happy, the sick people were happy, he was happy.

They discussed the details of getting to Nakuru and the expectation that they would probably have to take a hamper of food and a cold box of beers for the crew. The production assistant would see to that. The problem was that there might not be a restaurant up to the crew's standards in that direction. There were restaurants but some TV people did not think they were good enough.

'That's great,' the director said. 'It will be good to have got out of Nairobi to show we have really done the country. We'll be able to stop on the way and get some scenery shots too which should impress Mr and Mrs at home. Maybe some wildlife. What's the situation with the health minister for the next day?'

'When we left home,' the researcher said, 'we still didn't know whether the minister himself is on. But we've got a telex saying they'll put up someone anyway.'

'OK, keep on it, the location will be the same anyway. What about our prostitutes? Where are the most infected ones?'

'I've been looking for a nice infected one for you,' the researcher laughed. 'Look, there are two options. There are night clubs and discos basically around this area where we are now. Quite high-class prostitutes in Kenyan terms, maybe £25 a go.'

'That's more than I pay back home!' They all laughed. For some reason the commonplace that sex could be exchanged for money was always entertaining.

'But then there's Pumwani on the edge of Nairobi where they do it for between £1 and £2.50. Eighty-eight per cent are positive for the AIDS virus.'

'Great, let's go there. You got good contacts there, Jimmy?'

'I know many ladies there.'

'Bet you do. Great, that's it then, we'll do that on the afternoon of the third day, talk to a few girls. Maybe we'll get off in time to do some shopping that night. We fly back early the next day. Do you want to work out some call times with Jimmy?' he asked the PA. She and Jimmy began to work out a detailed schedule.

'Can we do an intro now?' the director asked the researcher.

'Can't it wait till the edit?' said the researcher, who was hoping to get to the swimming pool before dinner.

'It could. But I'm a professional and I like to know what I'm going for before I get it. I just want a form of words that I know I'm going in on. How many people are positive for the virus around here?'

'One to two per cent around here, three to four per cent in the western part of the country.'

'Mmm, and how many people in the country altogether?'

'Twenty million.'

'Look what about something like, we'll go for the lower figure to average it out.' He fiddled with a calculator, computing two per cent of 20,000,000. 'How about "Up to 400,000 people in Kenya now have the AIDS virus. As the tropical sun dips behind the slums of Pumwani the prostitutes with their deadly secret wait for new clients. Eighty-eight per cent of prostitutes here are infected yet the clients keep coming." And then we see a client go in a door, see?'

'Great, it's a winner.'

The hacks and the facts

An article titled 'AIDS in Africa' appeared in the *Guardian* on 2 February 1987 under the byline of Peter Murtagh. Two paragraphs ran:

Many of the truck drivers like nothing better than to round off a day's work by visiting a prostitute. Pumwani, a slum area on the edge of Nairobi, has two flat blocks where some 600 women service their needs for between £1 and £2.50. According to research, the women average up to 1000 partners a year.

In 1980 some of the prostitutes were tested for AIDS at their local sexually transmitted disease clinic. At that time, none was HIV positive. Three years later, fifty-three per cent were and now the figure is believed to be over eighty per cent.

Strong stuff. They must have a serious problem there.

A publication called the Panos Dossier appeared in November 1986. Supported by the Norwegian Red Cross, it claimed to report on 'AIDS and the Third World'. Under the heading 'AIDS Threatens Trucktown' is the following piece:

> In a Nairobi slum – let's call it Trucktown – over 600 women live in two decrepit-looking apartment compounds. They earn their money from the only employment they can find: prostitution.
>
> There are no fathers, no male wage-earners in Trucktown. The women earn about fifty US cents from each of their customers, who only come during the day. Many of the men are truck drivers passing through on their way to Mombasa. They stop for a 'tea break' and are soon on the road again.
>
> Each woman averages 1000 sexual partners a year. She suffers from sexually transmitted diseases, so she often visits the STD clinic. In 1980 the Trucktown women had their blood tested for the AIDS virus: none of them had it. They had never heard of AIDS.
>
> In 1983, they were tested again, and fifty-three per cent of them were carrying HIV. Now, over eighty per cent are HIV positive.

Notice any similarities? Of the many remarks which could be made about this, those of Richard and Rosalind Chirimuuta are particularly choice. The piece clearly shows Kenya's foremost position in medical research, they said, AIDS was only recognised in the United States in 1981 and the blood test introduced in 1984, but here was Kenya ahead of the world having identified the virus and introduced a blood test for antibodies in 1980.

Felix Konotey-Ahulu, the most sedulous of researchers, was unable to substantiate any of the inflated comments about AIDS in Kenya. He interviewed and in some cases worked with doctors, nurses, ministers of health, directors of medical services, research workers, ministers of religion, users of traditional medicine, taxi drivers, waiters and prostitutes. He visited sixteen African countries including those most affected by AIDS and he already had considerable experience of many of those countries.

As an antidote to wild exaggeration about African AIDS, see what Konotey-Ahulu wrote in *The Lancet* for 25 July 1987:

> If one judges the extent of the AIDS in Africa on an arbitrary scale from grade I (not much of a problem) to grade V (a catastrophe), in

my assessment AIDS is a problem (grade II) in only five (possibly six, since I was unable to obtain a visa for Zaire), of the countries where AIDS has occurred. Information I received from WHO (Congo Brazzaville), and from doctors I wrote to in other countries enabled me to grade the continent's problem in 1987. In no country is the AIDS problem consistently grade III (a great problem), nor ever grade IV (an extremely great problem) and in none can it be called a catastrophe (grade V). In Kenya, for instance, contrary to widespread reports I would rate AIDS in 1987 as grade I.

Gottlieb Monekosso, the director of the World Health Organization's regional office for Africa, supports this view. He remarked that AIDS figures tenth or lower on the list of African health problems. Most Africans are still getting sick and dying from diarrhoeal illnesses, measles, malaria and the other tropical diseases endemic in Africa. Of course, this could change, but AIDS has a long way to go before it is as serious a problem as tuberculosis.

Statistics are useful, as Carlyle points out, in as much as they can be used to stop ignorance from being foisted upon us. These are the AIDS cases, continent by continent, since the epidemic started to the end of 1987:

AIDS Cases Reported to WHO by Year as of 12 January 1988

	?	1979	1980	1981	1982	1983	1984	1985	1986	1987	1988	Total
Africa	1	0	0	0	3	14	82	206	2441	5946	0	8693
America	68	14	66	277	1054	3188	6267	11302	17090	17632	0	56958
Asia	0	0	1	0	1	8	4	29	54	127	0	224
Europe	8	0	4	16	72	218	578	1392	2635	3852	0	8775
Oceania	0	0	0	0	2	6	45	124	240	325	0	742
Total	77	14	71	293	1132	3434	6976	13053	22460	27882	0	75392

So as a continent Africa rates third out of five in the severity of its reported AIDS epidemic. America is by far the most severe with six and a half times the severity of the African situation.

Of course there could easily be under-reporting. It can be assumed that most AIDS cases in the USA are recorded; in Africa this may not be so. AIDS cases in Africa have, however, almost all been in population centres, particularly capital cities and large towns. Affected individuals may well have then travelled to their home villages to be ill with their families but from the start AIDS in Africa was an urban phenomenon – that is, it occurred among people who had access to VD clinics and hospital services.

Konotey-Ahulu, attempting to investigate extravagant claims about emergency hospital admissions for AIDS in Kenya, visited major hospitals and did ward rounds with consultants. 'I saw no AIDS admissions on two weekdays in February, but Dr Nelson Sewankambo informs me that on the worst occasion, out of 100 successive emergencies he would admit two or three with AIDS.'

Of course the possibility of under-reporting of AIDS cases is accepted, but there is also over-reporting. In an area where resources are scarce, with funding for AIDS projects being made available, other diseases might well find themselves being classified as AIDS cases. The wide parameters of the definition of AIDS in Africa as endorsed by the WHO does not help this. It was appreciated that a clinical case definition of AIDS was needed in a situation where diagnostic resources are limited. The provisional case definition for adults put out on 10 March 1986 was:

> Generalised Kaposi's sarcoma or cryptococcal meningitis are sufficient alone for a diagnosis of AIDS. Otherwise, at least two of the following major signs associated with one minor sign in the absence of other known causes of immunosuppression:
> *Major:* Loss of more than ten per cent of body weight
> Chronic diarrhoea for more than one month
> Prolonged fever for more than one month
> *Minor:* Persistent cough for more than one month
> General itchy skin rashes
> Recurrent shingles
> Oral thrush
> Progressive herpes sores
> Swollen lymph glands

There is therefore space for considerable over-estimation of AIDS cases even without involving HIV and alleged cases of HIV infection.

Konotey-Ahulu knows Africa and knows the African way of death. If tens of thousands are dying from AIDS, he says, where are the graves? Such questions are a far cry from a TV programme on AIDS in Africa which claimed one and a half million Africans might die from AIDS in the next five years.

Disease patterns from blood samples

Journalists were only able to make inflated claims about lifestyles and death in Africa because the HIV testers gave them the ammunition to do it. The central criticism is of double standards, of African and European patients being treated differently. Most importantly, AIDS cases – and high-risk individuals – in white countries are considered to be at risk because of what they do. They use drugs, they practise homosexual acts, they use contaminated blood products. Africans are considered at risk because of what they are, their racial makeup. African doctors and journalists have complained about this in vain.

Philip Ochieng commented in *New African*:

> The methods used to determine the spread of AIDS in the West and in Africa are vastly different. In the West the emphasis is on actual cases reported and projections based on lifestyles. In Africa a few people, mostly prostitutes, are rounded up and subjected to screening. Whenever AIDS *antibodies* are discovered, the medical boffins juggle their calculators and come up with figures that suggest half the entire nation is suffering from AIDS. If the same system of calculation was applied to California, the results might well indicate that every citizen there had not only contracted AIDS but had died from it.

This approach arose out of seroepidemiology – the taking of blood from as many people as possible to measure 'seropositivity', that is whether or not the people are HIV antibody-positive.

When the HIV antibody testing procedure became available in 1984, researchers made the journey to Africa, where they tested everyone they could find. 250 outpatients at a hospital in a remote area of eastern Zaire were studied and more than twelve per cent had antibodies against HIV but none had AIDS. In Kenya around the same time the number with antibodies went up to twenty-one per cent. This was the study which found one ethnic group, the Turkana, were showing fifty per cent seropositivity.

By the end of 1985 even the most fervent HIV enthusiasts admitted they had got it wrong: the tests were showing a 'false positive'. People were reacting as positive for the antibodies to the virus when the virus had never been near them. Probably the antibody test was reacting as positive to antibodies produced against something else – malaria was often suggested and as the research was done in the 'malaria belt' of sub-Saharan Africa (the area where AIDS is said to be rife) there is no doubt that many if not all the subjects would have come into contact with the parasite which causes malaria.

From the end of 1985 onwards, researchers were aware of the dangers of false positivity in Africa, though the damage, in implying Africa was over-run with disease carriers, was already done.

Nor did seroepidemiology cease. February 1987 found a number of researchers, including Max Essex, writing about the widespread appearance of antibodies to HIV and to HTLV-IV on the Ivory Coast 'despite the rarity of overt acquired immunodeficiency syndrome.'

So *Lancet* readers were treated to information about 12.9 per cent of prostitutes studied and 12.8 per cent of prisoners, for example, being antibody-positive to a fictitious virus. As has now been admitted, HTLV-IV was a laboratory contamination – the virus had never been near a human except the lab workers. It came from a macaque. All the subjects studied: the Tortiya prostitutes and Adzope prisoners and the Abidjan psychiatric patients were showing a false positive reaction.

The monkey sits at the centre of the AIDS story laughing like the mischievous monkey god in Eastern mythology.

Sero-archaeology

What makes the monkey so important? It is not that it gets AIDS after inoculation with HIV, for no laboratory animal does that. The monkey is not a model for human AIDS. The reason for the importance of the monkey is not that it elucidates a theory about AIDS, it is that the monkey fits in with an earlier theory.

Remember the days of HTLV-I, the 'leukaemia virus'. This virus was found in Japan, the Caribbean and Africa. Antibodies which reacted with the virus were found in African monkeys. When the viruses of these monkeys were examined, it was found they had some similarities to HTLV-I. The most similar strains were those from an African green monkey. Robert Gallo proposed the hypothesis that HTLV-I originated in Africa where it infected many species of primates, including humans. It reached the Americas along with the slave trade. It reached Japan by almost the same route; African slaves and monkeys were taken to Japan by Portuguese traders.

This is an amusing hypothesis which does nobody any harm. It cannot be proved either way but that is in the nature of historical theories. What did it have to do with AIDS? Robert Gallo had hypothesized that AIDS was caused by a virus which belonged to his HTLV family. He therefore extended the theory of an African origin direct from HTLV-I to HTLV-III. Max Essex, a supporter and collaborator of Robert Gallo's, enthusiastically set about demonstrating an African source for HTLV-III and this involved a study of non-human primates, in particular those which had been studied in connection with the earlier virus. When HTLV-III became known as HIV, it brought its intellectual baggage with it, including African origin.

Another section of the theory was the transmission from monkey to man in which the virus which did the monkey no harm was claimed to mutate into a virus which did harm man.

As the AIDS establishment was so convinced AIDS was a species crossover virus which had come from a monkey somewhere in Africa, it seemed a good idea to spend some research funds looking into the past of AIDS in Africa. How far back did the disease go?

In a process dubbed sero-archaeology, stored blood was examined. The most famous of these studies examined 1213 specimens, including some which had been stored since 1959. Eureka! One sample from 1959 gave a positive result. The authors, who again included the ubiquitous Max Essex, wrote: 'We have demonstrated that at least one individual from central Africa had been exposed to a virus similar to (HIV) more than a quarter of a century ago.'

Of course, there was no AIDS in the community from which this sample had been taken and in the absence of any further supportive information, and the presence of data contradicting it, it was allowed to sink into academic oblivion.

As Jonathan Mann, director of the World Health Organization's special programme on AIDS wrote:

[A] problem in testing old blood samples is that false positives can also occur if, for example, the frozen blood has thawed and then been refrozen. To make the situation even more complex, many Africans probably have relatively high levels of antibodies, proteins that signal the body's attempt to fight disease, in their blood, as a result of having other infections, such as malaria. These numerous antibodies tend to bond to one another and cause blood samples to become 'sticky', which may lead to false positive results with some tests.

Jonathan Mann additionally gave information on how the myth of an African origin for AIDS was given scientific respectability. In May 1984 the government of Zaire invited researchers from the Institute of Tropical Medicine in Antwerp, Belgium, and the US Centers for Disease Control to establish a long-time research project in collaboration with local clinicians and research scientists. Zaire was the first country to establish such a project. It was therefore the first country from which research papers were published and the first country to suffer media attention.

Mann remarks: 'This willingness had a disadvantage; for some time, the media thought that Zaire was the centre of the AIDS epidemic in Africa, or at least the most severely affected area. This mistake arose simply because good research from the Zairian project produced so many scientific publications.'

The African origin theory did not enjoy a Götterdämmerung in the conference halls of science, it died a slow death, failure to thrive rather than a battleaxe through the skull.

Seroepidemiology began to move against the African origin of AIDS theory when a West German team of researchers writing in *The Lancet* on 26 October 1985 reported on serum collected from 3159 African patients and found only two showed positive when subjected to the most sensitive tests. As this sera was collected between 1981 and the date of testing, it suggested that HIV 'was rare in Africa until recently and still is rare in much of the continent'.

When the results of a much larger study were published in the *British Medical Journal* on 27 September 1986, the results were even more striking. 6015 samples were tested, collected between 1976 and 1984 in nine African countries. By the most commonly used antibody test, the ELISA, ten per cent were antibody-positive. By more sensitive methods four of the samples were found to be positive, a rate of less than one per one thousand and, as the authors noted, 'lower than that found in German blood donors'.

This evidence cannot be fully acceptable to those who say HIV does not cause AIDS. It is valuable, however, in that carrying antibodies to HIV is an indication of having come into contact with the sort of behaviour which predisposes a person to develop AIDS. HIV can be taken in Africa, therefore, as a 'marker of promiscuity' as it is elsewhere. The German team's work supports this position, though of course they consider HIV to be a direct cause of AIDS.

In terms of promiscuity and the spread of AIDS, the Germans note the absence of HIV positivity in village communities – promiscuous sexual behaviour is difficult if not impossible in a traditional African village. 'Risk groups have been identified as urban-dwelling, wealthy, mobile, and promiscuous heterosexual men, their wives and children and women prostitutes.'

When AIDS cases are examined epidemiologically it is obvious that the poor, rural Africans do not figure as victims unless they have been in contact with wealthier city dwellers. AIDS in Africa originated in Africans with a history of foreign travel. Indeed, hospitals in Belgium, France and the UK have cared for Africans with AIDS since the earliest days of the epidemic. It is a tiny minority of Africans who get sick at home and then decide to go to Europe for treatment.

It seems most likely that foreigners visiting the centres of prostitution in Africa took AIDS to the continent by having sex with the more expensive prostitutes. These were precisely the prostitutes employed by high-class Africans. The role of homosexual prostitution in Africa will probably forever remain murky. Homosexuality is frowned upon severely in most African communities, if not all of them. African homosexuals suffer in an atmosphere similar to that of the nineteenth century in Western countries. They are unlikely to admit to homosexuality. Homosexuals are likely to be married and so spread a disease homosexually contracted into the heterosexual community. Homosexual prostitution, including homosexual prostitution with Westerners, might well be practised by men who have bowed to community pressure to marry. Additionally, the situation may be similar to that in Haiti where impoverished heterosexual men are driven to homosexual prostitution as a means of keeping their families fed.

The international epidemiology of AIDS also supports the theory that the Westerners gave it to the Africans rather than vice versa. Richard and Rosalind Chirimuuta in *Aids, Africa and Racism* remark on 'the absence of AIDS in Angola, Mozambique and Namibia, the former two countries sharing borders with "high incidence" countries. All three of these war-torn states have had little contact with Americans or Western Europeans since the beginning of the AIDS epidemic, whilst there has been considerably more contact with nationals of the AIDS affected neighbouring states.' If AIDS spread from Africans, it should have spread to other African countries at the same time as or before the spread to Western countries.

The nail in the coffin of the African origin theory came at the international conference on AIDS in Africa, held in Naples in October 1987. Luc Montagnier, the man who discovered HIV-1 and HIV-2 said the evidence for an African origin was 'very weak . . . Maybe we should look at another part of the world'. If there were an African origin, there should have been a reservoir of infection among some tribe or other, presumably the one where the momentous monkey bite had first occurred, but no such reservoir has been discovered. Perhaps darkest Africa has not yielded up her secret or, as Montagnier feels more likely, perhaps there was no secret to yield up.

The African origin theory has been hard to abandon. It was attractive for AIDS theorists to think of a horrifying disease to shock the world being brewed up in a jungle in darkest Africa as a result of some kind of grotesque congress between man and monkey. In fact all the evidence, whether we look at cases of AIDS or of HIV infection, is that the Africans were just like everyone else in this story, just ordinary people trying to live their lives in peace when they found themselves with this disease in their midst and they knew not whence it had come.

Perhaps the swan-song of the African origin theory has been the monkey food research. This was work published in *Trends in Ecology and Evolution* in December 1987 by researchers who wondered why the African green monkey is infected with a virus similar to HIV but does not develop AIDS. Of the range of reasons why this might occur, some are complicated and some are very simple indeed. The reason these researchers chose to investigate was that perhaps something in the African green monkey's diet protects it from developing AIDS. To put it another way: 'Natural selection may well have favoured those monkeys that included anti-viral substances in their diet.' Presumably there would have been no research grant forthcoming for simply saying that the presence of something like HIV in healthy animals suggested HIV was not a deadly pathogen.

AIDS in Africa

Apart from the exaggerations and mere inventions, the facts of AIDS in Africa exist. While medical care is limited in many areas, it is inconceivable that a disease with such marked symptoms – disabling oral thrush, for example – could be overlooked for long. An epidemic has been progressing in Africa perhaps at a faster rate than in the West. Its characteristics are dissimilar in that chronic diarrhoea is often the first and most obvious symptom, but the lung parasite Pneumocystis carinii and the skin cancer Kaposi's sarcoma also make their appearance as in the West.

Much has been made of the higher level of heterosexual transmission in Africa than in the West. If we exclude the homosexual cases from figures for, say, the US, the ratio of female to male AIDS victims begins to even up.

To be more explicit: it is foolish to compare American figures, in which we know homosexual intercourse is a significant factor, with African figures, in which it almost certainly is not.

Among some of the victims malnutrition, which is a known cause of immune depression, might well contribute to susceptibility to AIDS. But most of the early cases were not poor. There are other fragmentary explanations – condom use is not extensive in Africa for a variety of reasons. Prostitutes failing to use condoms, which are covered in a slight lubricant, might be more open to vaginal trauma which would predispose to infection. Prostitutes may also be less frequently using lubricant creams than their Western sisters. Genital herpes and ulcerative genital conditions have also been suggested as being particularly likely to hasten the spread of AIDS.

Traditional African healing techniques, particularly those involving cutting the body and inserting some kind of herb under the skin, have been criticised as a method by which AIDS can be spread. Far more likely is that new medical methods imported from the West have been a means of spreading AIDS. 'Injectionists' sell injections of medicines or, doubtless, coloured water, from bar to bar. They are hardly equipped to sterilise the needles.

Disease eradication programmes have also been implicated in the spread of AIDS, a particular finger being pointed at the smallpox eradication programme of the late nineteen-seventies where poor hygienic procedures may have been responsible for the re-use of contaminated needles on large groups of people.

Antibiotics can be immune-suppressive. The over-use of antibiotics in Third World countries has long been an issue among campaigners for rational drugs policies. They are concerned that the poor should have appropriate medicines to their needs but also that repeated small doses of powerful drugs can allow the pathogen they are aimed at combating to build up a resistance.

Whatever the specific cause of the pattern of the epidemic in Africa, it is certain that the inappropriate application of technology designed to detect HIV antibodies did the continent a great deal of harm. This is particularly depressing if HIV has little to do with AIDS even when it is accurately detected.

There is more than national (or continental) pride at stake when countries are stigmatised as being plague-ridden. An AIDS scare based on faulty epidemiology could severely reduce the income from tourism in countries where there are few major industries. When an industry like tourism begins to collapse, a knock-on effect runs through the whole workforce from the bank clerks and air stewards to the fruit pickers and street sellers.

Additionally there is the problem of travel to countries where work is in more plentiful supply. South Africa, never known for its enlightened social policies, has declared it will refuse admission to workers from other countries who are HIV positive. Thus faulty blood testing, based on what is probably a misapprehension about the relationship between HIV and AIDS, is condemning these men and the families they support to hunger.

Nine

Finance

Following the money

AT THE END of 1987 Washington gossip was rich with the news of Robert Gallo's intention to leave the National Institutes of Health and set up an AIDS institute which would be run in association with Johns Hopkins University in Baltimore.

The proposal for the institute was backed by the brothers David and Isaac Blech who have made, and invested, big money in biotechnology. The new institute would have involved money from private investors, the insurance industry (which has lost millions in payments to young men who were good insurance risks until they got AIDS) and the Blech company Nova Pharmaceuticals.

Other Blech companies include Genetic Systems, DNA Plant Technology and Cambridge BioScience. Cambridge BioScience produces HIV testing kits and a considerable number of shares in it are owned by AIDS researchers and Gallo collaborators Max Essex and William Haseltine.

The involvement of AIDS researchers in AIDS businesses could be pursued with innuendo and research showing international links but such a pursuit would not, in the end, tell us more than we already know. The AIDS researchers believed in what they were doing and if businesses were being set up on the basis of their work, they may as well make some money themselves out of it. Some might well consider it a scandal that scientists should have such a pecuniary interest in the success of their theories but it would also be considered a scandal if scientists lived modestly while business people enjoyed the fruits of their labours. If Essex and Haseltine hadn't been sufficiently committed to their research to invest in it themselves, how could they have expected others to have done so?

Haseltine and Essex deny that their business investments have affected their work and as we would doubtless receive a similar denial from all other AIDS researchers with their own money backing the HIV theory, the issue of individual investments had better rest there.

The point is, anyway, not that individual greed shores up questionable theories, but that science does not function in a vacuum divorced from the pressures and structures which make up the society in which it works.

HIV was discovered in an atmosphere in which filing the patent application for the procedures which would lead to the test kits was as important as publication in the scientific journals. Once the French and Americans had entered into a three-year dispute about who came first, how could they back down on the central question of whether the virus causes the disease?

There was always a lot at stake – national prestige, personal prestige and big, big money. The market for the test kits was estimated at $100 million a year. AIDS was a business with a big future.

The Technology Management Group, which analyses investment trends, issued a report in July 1986 predicting that the world market for products to treat, diagnose and prevent AIDS is likely to be $3.1 billion in 1996. They noted 2034 different companies and organisations working on the AIDS business including 521 doing basic research, 381 on drug treatments and 155 producing diagnostics – the good old testing kits.

Nearly forty drugs are being tested in AIDS. Their success or failure makes a considerable difference to the balance sheet. Du Pont shares shot up after the news leaked out about the wonder drug Ampligen. It had been tested on just ten people.

Private investment is dwarfed when compared to the huge sums governments can hand over. The total AIDS budget in the US was $28.7 million in 1983 and $61.5 million in 1984. By 1 April 1987 President Reagan would be announcing AIDS to be 'public health enemy number one' and saying the administration was spending $766 million on AIDS research that year with an intended amount in excess of $1 billion in 1988. Some critics said this money, particularly in the early days, was money which had been allocated to other programmes and which was only being diverted to AIDS; it was not a new budget.

It was like the old days of cancer research: any establishment which had an idea on HIV could have a grant to work on it. Theoretically, a large investment in AIDS research should lead to sufficient numbers of people becoming familiar enough with the disease for some to realise that it cannot be caused by HIV or cannot be caused by HIV alone. Unfortunately, all the work is calculated to reinforce the notion that HIV alone causes AIDS. Peter Duesberg has actually dealt with these grant applications. He said:

> I was asked to serve on the California task force for AIDS. This is state money that is all of a sudden available for basic research on AIDS. It's not available for cancer or any other of the well known problems of mankind, just AIDS.
>
> Of the twenty applications assigned to me, twenty of them proposed to study this virus as the cause of AIDS. Not one of them even considered the question of whether the virus is indeed the cause of AIDS: is there sufficient proof of it or could something else be analysed for study?
>
> People come up with a hundred thousand or two hundred thousand dollar projects per year and they get the money for it. A number of laboratories that have been quiet until recently are now very active and have a lot of money to study and sequence a dormant virus in cell culture.
>
> HIV has become big business not just for laboratories, it has also been a boost for the scientific journals and for the press and for politicians. It has attracted money and attention to science.

The quest for a vaccine

Vaccination is the only contribution of virology to human health and happiness to date, and it is understandable that the quest for a vaccine should have been the first thought of virus hunters once they had found HIV.

There are some central difficulties in constructing a vaccine in the laboratory. Classically the principle is that healthy people are injected with a tiny number of the micro-organisms they are to be protected against. Sometimes not the organisms themselves but the toxin ('poison') they produce is injected. This stimulates the immune system: the invader is identified and the T4 cells summon B cells to produce antibodies which neutralise the enemy. When that attack is over the T8 or killer T cells destroy infected body cells and thus cleanse the system of the invader completely. Soon the only evidence that there has been an invasion is stored in the memory T cells which retain a chemical 'memory' of the invader. Whenever the same micro-organism, or a significantly similar one, attacks after this, the memory T cells instruct the other parts of the immune system how to respond. It is a sort of chemical 'learned response'.

The problem with HIV in this context is that it does not produce a toxin which could be used to stimulate an immune response without causing the disease. As a latent virus, it doesn't seem to do anything. Moreover, there is already profuse antibody production against HIV. As has been noted, it is one of the paradoxes of HIV that the higher the level of antibodies against it in the blood, the more at risk a person is of going on to develop AIDS. This is, at any rate, the claim of those who believe HIV alone causes AIDS.

It is possible to put some of the proteins from the coat of HIV on to an inert chemical. Injected into a person who has not come into contact with HIV before, it triggers the immune system to begin producing antibodies against HIV. Then when the real HIV comes along, the memory T cells will recognise it and produce antibodies before it can enter the T4 cell, which is its favoured home. This, at any rate, is the theory.

The 'mutagenicity' of the protein coat of the virus is one of the greatest problems here. Basically this just means it keeps changing. Part of the means by which viruses survive is that they go through a series of tiny mutations, so the antibody against this year's influenza virus, for example, will not protect against next year's influenza virus. If it is successful in its survival strategy, the micro-organism will have changed just sufficiently to get past the antibodies which were produced for the previous incarnation of the virus.

HIV is such a virus, according to some researchers, and there are different strains of HIV isolated from different patients even in the same city.

There is something of a rush in the scientific community to lay claim to bits of HIV in the hope that the bit they have staked a claim to will form part of an eventual vaccine against HIV. Thus in February 1988 Max Essex and his co-researchers at Harvard University won a patent on gp 120 (glycoprotein 120), part of the envelope or coat of HIV.

Since 1977 scientists have been able to claim a patent on forms of life they have 'discovered'. Once again in the AIDS research story the word 'hubris' springs to mind.

A major problem with the viral research programme is, of course, that if the virus does not cause AIDS, a huge sum of money will be spent on a vaccine against a virus no more damaging than cytomegalovirus. It also ought to be remembered that all vaccination programmes carry the risk of some individuals reacting badly against the vaccine. A vaccine, particularly for mass use, has to be as near perfectly safe as possible. Additionally, there is a major ethical problem of testing. How do you test a vaccine which is supposed to confer protection against AIDS? Inject them with the vaccine, then give them a syringe full of blood from an AIDS patient? The lack of an animal model for AIDS has bedevilled AIDS research from the start.

Even if a successful vaccine were to be produced, it is uncertain what the rewards would be. Dino Dina heads vaccine research at the Chiron Corporation, one of the seventy-five companies worldwide working on a vaccine against HIV. He said:

> The financial rewards for a vaccine like this are variable and probably determined both by psychological and political considerations.
>
> If you were to be the only manufacturer of a vaccine of this type and if your target population were the high risk individuals and some lower risk individuals like health care workers, then you could expect to have sizeable markets and to be able to sell your vaccine for relatively high prices.
>
> But if this were to turn into a competitive business and many manufacturers were on the market and if this were then adopted for childhood vaccination through government agencies, it could very rapidly then become a commodity business, very similar to polio virus vaccination and other childhood vaccinations where there is essentially no money to be made.

Neutralising antibodies and research grants

Part of the way scientists have tried to overcome the paradox of the production of antibodies in HIV-infected people who then go on to develop AIDS is to question the nature of the antibodies produced. The reason the HIV antibodies do not prevent a person from developing AIDS is, they say, not because HIV does not cause AIDS but because the antibodies don't work well enough.

This question of the neutralising and the non-neutralising antibodies was proposed by Abraham Karpas of the University of Cambridge in 1985. He said it was possible that the reason why most people who have HIV antibodies do not have AIDS is that the antibodies genuinely are doing their job and holding back the infection. So why do some people die from AIDS even though they are producing antibodies prolifically? Their antibodies are ineffective, they are non-neutralising antibodies, Karpas's thought runs.

This may be a rather tortuous line of reasoning but at least Abraham Karpas was prepared to attack the questions head on; less daring researchers were pretending there was no problem. His early research led to some confidence in his ideas, so he applied to the UK's Medical Research Council for a grant of £116,000 in 1986.

The rejection said 'that this was not a well-designed application' and that it 'lacked originality'. In a letter to the *Listener*, Abraham Karpas complained when an application for £1,000,000 from Robin Weiss of the Institute of Cancer Research was successful despite what Karpas felt to be its similarity to his own proposal.

Abraham Karpas has been described as an abrasive and outspoken personality. He is certainly not an establishment voice. He feels that he has been excluded from research funding, journals and conferences.

Karpas did succeed in mounting his study after receiving funding from Medicorp of the US in return for development rights to any new procedure which results. The HIV testing kit which Karpas developed has also been sold, to Fuji Chemical, to fund research. It should not be thought that business interests invariably act to the detriment of science; the criticism of the early days of AIDS research is not that business was a possibility in the future but that the business angle was allowed to play too great a part too early on.

Peer review

The influence of the journals and the peer-review system is another pressure on science which has money at the back of it. The major journals like *Science* and *Nature* have vast sums backing them. The medical journals have almost exclusively pharmaceutical advertising. There might be occasions where the weight of advertising and other moneys channeled into a journal make its staff tend towards corruption but this is not really the problem. The problem is that the weight of establishment backing for the journals makes them always tend towards orthodoxy. Orthodoxy strangles original thought.

The peer-review system, in which articles are sent by the journal to 'peers' of the original researcher, determines the direction research is going to take. A writer of a paper will ensure it is something which is acceptable to the journal – it must not stray too far from orthodoxy but must make a contribution which is a genuine advance on what is already known. The journal editor will send it to a specialist in the same field who will also be involved in research. He will either reject it or accept it or, more likely, make suggestions based on his own theories which would 'correct' erroneous assumptions made in the paper. This means he would urge it further into line with his own thought, with the orthodox view.

This same person would sit on funding committees and applications for appointments at scientific research establishments. He would exert the same conservative influence there, unless he were a most unusual person.

Once, twenty or thirty years ago, scientific research was a quiet activity, undertaken far away from the public gaze; now researchers become media stars.

The public demands stars and it is natural for humans to enjoy the respect of their co-workers, their readers, their TV audience. The inducement is first to publish more than your rivals, almost regardless of quality, then to popularise your work in the journals for general readers, then to appear on the TV chat show as an expert on your branch of science, on science in general, on life.

The race for first publication, massaging the data to make it fit, the race for the scientific award, these are not essentially financial yearnings but they are avaricious nevertheless.

The anti-virals

The Wellcome Foundation, formerly a charitable trust, became a public company in February 1986. Its shares traded on the London Stock Exchange at 120p. Within a year the shares had reached 450p. Behind it was their AIDS drug, universally known as AZT despite their efforts to familiarise the medical profession with their brand name: Retrovir.

This was for a long time a drug looking for a disease to treat. It was first isolated from herring sperm by Jerome Horwitz at the Michigan Cancer Foundation in 1961, then synthesised by him in 1964. It was promising but eventually unsuccessful as an anti-cancer agent.

It was not patented because there was no use for it at that time. Wellcome's US subsidiary was screening known agents for anti-bacterial properties in the early nineteen-eighties when Sam Broder, working independently at the National Cancer Institute in the US, discovered it had properties which inhibited HIV *in vitro* – in the test tube.

The National Cancer Institute turned over its data and technology to Wellcome. Wellcome applied to the US regulatory authority, the Food and Drug Administration, for 'orphan drug' status for the compound which they received in July 1985. This was a right conferred under a piece of humane legislation designed to encourage the development of drugs which would not benefit a great many patients but were nevertheless capable of being produced. Normally drug companies can only afford to produce drugs which will be used by a large number of people, thus giving an adequate return on investment. Under orphan drug rules, the company involved agrees to produce the drug and enjoys seven years' exclusive marketing rights plus tax incentives. Additionally, the FDA sets no limit on the price of the drug.

Herring sperm is in short supply so Wellcome made a deal with the drug company Pfizer to supply it exclusively with synthetic herring sperm extract, called thymidine.

Trials started in July 1985 with 282 patients with AIDS or the 'pre-AIDS' condition called AIDS-Related Complex. The study was intended to last twenty-four weeks but at the end of only seventeen weeks it was discontinued.

The reason was that AZT reduced the death rates in the 145 patients who took it – only one of them died. In the group which was being compared, taking an inactive placebo, 19 out of 137 died. The AZT patients were also doing much better, they were suffering fewer opportunistic infections.

This type of trial, the 'double-blind, placebo-controlled' trial, is the philosophers' stone of medical research – it turns base theories into gold. If you have a drug which is successful in a trial of this type, it is a money-spinner. A double-blind placebo-controlled trial is almost as good as you can get in terms of fact which will convince research scientists, physicians and the public.

The principle is that all 'operator error' must be removed from the trial by dint of ensuring no one knows whether an active drug is being given to a patient or a 'placebo' – a harmless capsule which looks like the active drug. Not only must the patients be unaware, the doctors giving the medicine must also be ignorant of which patients are taking the drug. If they were not, they would betray, albeit unconsciously, this information to the patient and the patient would react differently – more hopefully if he knew he was on the drug.

John Lauritsen, writing in the *New York Native*, conducted a remarkable examination of this trial in which he pointed out areas in which the trial became 'unblinded', thereby seriously calling into question its results.

Initially there was a difference in taste between the placebo and the AZT. People with AIDS are, understandably, obsessed with their medication and spend a great deal of time comparing treatments. Very early in the trial it was clear to many whether they were getting AZT or the placebo. This taste difference was soon corrected but the damage was done.

Another way patients became aware whether they were on placebo or AZT was by taking their tablets to analysis. Finding they were on placebo would certainly decrease their chances of long-term survival. The one thing sure to be lethal in a seriously ill patient is to give up hope.

People with AIDS maintain a close, supportive community in those cities where the disease is widespread. Some of the people in the AZT trial pooled and shared out their medication so they all received at least some AZT. Some patients continued with the use of drugs illegally shipped from Mexico.

For these reasons, the results were flawed from the start. Additionally, the physicians were never 'blinded' – they were always aware of which patients were on AZT and which on placebo because of damage to the bone marrow (and therefore the blood cells) of patients using AZT. Its side effects gave it away.

Other criticisms of the trial were that because of the early termination of the trial, only fifteen patients finished the full twenty-four-week protocol, out of a total of 282. Twenty-four weeks was a short time, anyway, in which to test a drug which may be in clinical use for years of a patient's life. Cutting the trial short made statistical analysis difficult, as did changes in the method of notation midway through the trial when forms for noting patients' symptoms were changed over. The original ten-point form noting symptoms 'often associated with HIV infection' were withdrawn and replaced by a thirty-three-item 'AIDS related signs and symptoms' sheet.

Furthermore, as Lauritsen remarks:

> The death rate in the AZT group is suspiciously low when compared with other trials of AZT. After the 'double-blind, placebo-controlled' study was terminated, all patients were informed which treatment they had been receiving, and were offered the option of receiving AZT. A total of 227 patients accepted the offer, and continued or began to receive AZT.
>
> AZT no longer prevented patients from dying. In the twenty-one weeks of the 'open label' trial, ten per cent of the patients died. Curiously, not only deaths but also opportunistic infections increased in the original AZT group as soon as the first study was terminated. There is no good explanation why this should be so.

Regardless of the inadequacies of the trial, AZT is efficacious to some limited degree and the rush for it started.

At $1.88 per capsule with patients taking twelve capsules a day, the cost worked out at $8200 a year for every patient. Wellcome was enjoying a good return on this orphan drug. It would still, however, take them a long time to recover the money they had spent on its research and development. Stock market analysts reckon that if it is still the only AIDS drug available by 1989, Wellcome will have reaped profits of more than $130 million.

But there were problems. AZT is not, and has never been claimed to be, a cure for AIDS. Patients continued to die, they just took longer on AZT. Damage to the bone marrow meant frequent blood transfusions.

Other side effects such as confusion and bleeding from the anus may well have been effects of AIDS and not of AZT, but they were hardly evidence of an effective drug.

It is difficult to tell why AZT has its, admittedly limited, effectiveness against AIDS. It could be that HIV causes AIDS and that AZT is effective against HIV. This is possible but it is characteristic of the strait-jacket mentality which the HIV theory encourages that it is the only possibility which has been examined by those with the equipment to carry out appropriate tests. It could well be that AZT is having a real effect on a number of microbes including, because it happens to be there, HIV.

AZT certainly stops DNA replication which makes it rather more like aiming a shotgun at the body than a surgical laser. Described as an 'anti-metabolite', it stops the metabolism of HIV but also of many other things including the cells themselves. Hence the blood deficiencies which accompany its use.

Wellcome accepts this but says the doses required to stop cell DNA production are one hundred times greater than those required to stop reverse transcriptase production, which is what inhibits the HIV.

Wellcome's prescribing information is admirably candid on the level of clinical ignorance about the drug, which they refer to in this instance by its generic name of zidovudine:

> The relationship between *in vitro* susceptibility of HIV to zidovudine and the inhibition of HIV replication in man or clinical response to therapy has not been established. In vitro sensitivity results vary greatly depending upon the time between virus infection and zidovudine treatment, the particular assay used, the cell type employed, and the laboratory performing the test. In addition, the methods currently used to establish virologic responses in clinical trials may be relatively insensitive in detecting changes in the quantities of actively replicating HIV or reactivation of these viruses.

This last sentence means we are back to the original problem which Duesberg drew out so perceptively: if there is so little HIV in the body of an AIDS patient, if it is so inactive, how can we be sure it is ever doing anything? If we cannot even detect it in most cases when a person is ravaged with sickness, how can we expect to detect the changes in this virus alleged to be made by AZT?

AZT is a biochemically active substance and we know some of the micro-organisms against which it is active *in vitro*. Many gut bacteria which are a feature of AIDS are capable of being inhibited by AZT: Shigella which causes dysentery; Salmonella which causes gastro-enteritis and typhoid in two of its manifestations. Others causing disease given the right opportunity and conditions are Escherichia, Klebsiella, Enterobacter and Citrobacter. The parasite Giardia lamblia is also inhibited *in vitro.*

AZT crosses the blood brain barrier, separating nerve tissue from the bloodstream. It shares this capability with several micro-organisms known to infect AIDS patients including HIV, Toxiplasma gondii, Mycobacterium tuberculosis, cytomegalovirus and the syphilis pathogen Treponema pallidum.

It is likely that AZT has widespread anti-viral properties and its action involves holding back a number of micro-organisms and allowing the AIDS patient's body a chance to fight back.

David Goldmeier at the Praed Street clinic in London, who has been looking into the role of syphilis in 'AIDS dementia' notes that this condition is often relieved by AZT. 'It could be that because AZT decreases the viral load, this gives the white blood cells enough respite to cope with the treponemes .' That is, Treponema pallidum is causing neurosyphilis, the AZT holds back the viruses and allows the immune system to concentrate on the syphilis.

Anecdotal reports suggest that positive attitude, exercise and nutritious diet have as much success in extending the lives of AIDS patients as any therapeutic treatment yet known and also offer a better quality of life in those last remaining months than drug regimes can.

Other anti-virals

There are stories well worth telling about other anti-viral drugs being tested for use on AIDS patients but they have only a tangential connection with the question of whether HIV causes the disease. The discussion about how Dideoxycytidine, HPA-23, Ribavirin or AL-721 claim to combat AIDS would be only a rehearsal of arguments already put about AZT's alleged anti-AIDS activity.

In terms of the interaction between business, science and national prestige, it is worth noting the continued criticisms of the US authorities for allegedly giving favoured treatment to particular drugs at the expense of equally promising others. In particular it is claimed that the Food and Drug Administration which licenses medicines is dragging its feet over licensing treatments like Foscarnet because it is a foreign drug – in this case Swedish.

In June 1986 the US Congress awarded $141 million to fund a nationwide programme to test new AIDS treatments. Two thousand patients were supposed to be enrolled during the first year. After one year only 845 patients had been enrolled, 90 per cent of them in trials involving AZT.

Ten

Endgame

Scientific method?

SCIENTISTS DILIGENTLY PUSH forward the frontiers of knowledge, the occasional flash of inspiration speeding the slow progress of lab work. A theory is created and tested, the results look promising. They are published and other laboratories duplicate the work out of a sense of scientific cameraderie. Work pushes forward with publication at each step until finally the theory is vindicated and the scientist enjoys the applause of colleagues and public accolades.

A total fiction, of course. Science proceeds like any other area of human endeavour, with hard work, idling, corner cutting, jealousy, the deceitful padding of results to accommodate previously held views and the premature announcement of findings to be greeted with back-biting in the professional press.

To believe that science is in some peculiar way 'rational' or above the petty concerns which bedevil the human race is as absurd as believing that journalists are purveyors of the truth or lawyers vendors of justice. Of course, there is some validity in these statements: some truth is forthcoming and some justice available from journalistic and legal enterprises. But this is hardly the whole story. A young person does not have to be very advanced into adolescence before realising that there are other factors acting on professionals beside the abstract notions of truth or justice of which the average lawyer or journalist might not think from one week to the next. Remuneration, position in a hierarchy, the pressure to get results, obeisance to traditional values, skill and personal beliefs are all factors in professional life and scientists have no immunity.

The Austrian philosopher Paul Feyerabend, in criticising the theory of scientific 'method' as a realistic description of what actually happens in scientific development, gives an unintentional commentary on what happened in the quest for HIV.

Eschewing thinkers who claim that theories of method follow from the observation of scientific practice, Feyerabend demonstrates in *Against Method* that scientific inquiries do not and never have proceeded according to 'scientific method'. Indeed, even two of the most successful scientists, Galileo and Newton, were masters of deceit and the presentation of selected truths. While it is easiest and most interesting to see this in the case of great scientists of the past, it is also true that their contemporaries behaved in a like manner in defending theories which have not been passed down to us. Feyerabend considers science has made a mistake in divorcing scientific practice from the history of science and the philosophy of science. Scientists can only move towards the future if they have a comprehension of the randomness of past discoveries and the theories which informed them.

Feyerabend criticises the 'consistency condition' which insists that new ideas agree with accepted ideas. A perfect example of this in practice is the discovery that some antibiotics work against AIDS. The scientists who suggest that because antibiotics have only been known to work against bacteria in the past, this discovery suggests a bacterial cause for AIDS, are cold-shouldered out of the scientific community. The bacterial theory does not comply with the condition that a new theory must keep step with accepted ideas – in this case that AIDS is caused by a virus.

Other scientists who made a similar discovery about the efficacy of some antibiotics in AIDS patients, however, kept to the consistency condition by declaring that they had found an antibiotic which had this surprising anti-viral action, unlike all others of its class. Thou good and faithful servants.

This demand for consistency does not only abandon facts because they do not fit the theory, it abandons new theories which might be better suited to the facts. As Feyerabend says: 'It eliminates a theory or hypothesis not because it disagrees with the facts; it eliminates it because it disagrees with another theory, with a theory, moreover, whose confirming instances it shares. It therefore makes the as yet untested part of that theory a measure of validity.' In this case the 'untested part' is the link between the virus and AIDS. If the virus causes AIDS, then removing the virus will cure the AIDS. This has yet to be demonstrated. The antibiotics remove something and 'cure' (perhaps for a limited period) the disease. A proposition based on these facts is attacked with reference to an untested theory about the link between the virus and AIDS. To continue with the quote: 'The only difference between such a measure and a more recent theory is age and familiarity. Had the younger theory been there first, then the consistency condition would have worked in its favour. "The first adequate theory has a right of priority over equally adequate aftercomers.'"

Feyerabend accepts that we must follow the theories which we find interesting rather than those we find boring. As Peyton Rous said: 'Since what one thinks determines what one does . . . it is as well to think something.' There will, and should be, a theory. It is what then happens with competing theories as information starts to accrue which supports the chosen theory that Feyerabend criticises.

> Now assume that the pursuit of the chosen theory has led to successes, and that the theory has explained, in a satisfactory manner, circumstances that had been unintelligible for quite some time. This gives empirical support to an idea which to start with seemed to possess only this advantage: it was interesting and intriguing. The commitment to the theory will now be reinforced, and the attitude toward alternatives will become less tolerant. Now if it is true . . . that many facts become available only with the help of alternatives, then the refusal to consider them will result in the elimination of potentially refuting facts as well. More especially, it will eliminate facts whose discovery would show the complete and irreparable inadequacy of the theory.

In the case of AIDS and the HIV theory the way this works is that people with AIDS are simply considered to be people with HIV.

In most cases in the US, for example, whence the bulk of the world's cases come, there is no check for HIV. From the Centers for Disease Control's own figures, since 1985 less than seven per cent of AIDS cases in New York and San Francisco have been tested for HIV. There is no information which would support or refute the theory that another pathogen could be causing this disease – the HIV theory has simply swept such information to one side. Of course, there is no information to support the HIV theory either, for the same reason, but as it is so fully accepted as a matter of faith that HIV causes AIDS, no supporting information is required.

Once scientists are convinced of a proposition, it is extraordinarily difficult to get them to budge from it, despite the weight of conflicting fact. Feyerabend quotes Barrow, Isaac Newton's teacher and predecessor at Cambridge, commenting on an observation which challenged a theory with new fact: 'For me, neither this nor any other difficulty shall have so great an influence on me, as to make me renounce that which I know to be manifestly agreeable to reason.'

This could be the motto of AIDS scientists but, more appositely, of all those scientists and clinicians who are not even familiar with the papers covering the original work done on HIV, but accept the alleged causal relationship between virus and disease on trust.

Feyerabend congratulates Barrow on even being prepared to accept there are difficulties. 'The usual procedure is to forget the difficulties, never to talk about them, and to proceed as if the theory were without fault.'

He also comments on the way the language of observation is allowed to merge with the subject being observed so the theory becomes the fact. Thus Gallo argued for renaming AIDS 'HTLV-III disease'. This of course presupposes a link between disease and virus. AIDS is now sometimes referred to as 'HIV infection' or 'HIV disease'. Remember how the title of Joe Sonnabend's journal was changed from *AIDS Research*, which could be about anything to do with AIDS, to *AIDS and Human Retrovirus Research*, which presupposed the cause.

The tenacity with which scientists cleave to a chosen theory put one in mind of religion rather than empirically verifiable knowledge. New fact is forever incorporated into an old theory, the theory being reshaped to accommodate it. AIDS was characterised by a decline in the level of T4 cells, an essential part of the immune system. Robert Gallo declared AIDS must be caused by a virus which was part of his HTL family of viruses. Therefore it was believed that a virus like Gallo's original two gets into the T4 cells and kills them.

Actually it is now clear that HIV is not part of Gallo's family of viruses and it doesn't kill T4 cells directly by getting into a T4 cell and killing it from inside. OK, said the HIV supporters, it must cause AIDS in some other way.

HIV was said to cause AIDS in up to one hundred per cent of people in five years. Five years later HIV was widespread but deaths from AIDS did not correspond to the HIV figures. This is, the HIV supporters say, because it does not kill in one hundred per cent of cases but seventy per cent or fifty per cent or less. And it does not kill in five years, it will take eight years or longer. This is why the phrase 'moving the goalposts' is so apposite: all evidence which undermines the original theory is dealt with by altering the precepts of the original theory, not by examining it with a mind to abandoning it if it did not fit with the facts.

Helga Rübsamen-Waigmann of the Georg-Speyer-Haus, Frankfurt, is quoted by Duesberg for work she did which found HIV in the T4 cells of only eighty-eight out of ninety-one AIDS patients by the most assiduous methods of laboratory analysis – evidence that HIV is not necessary for AIDS, according to Duesberg.

Rübsamen-Waigmann puts it differently. She had looked for HIV in T cells and had looked for it in the central nervous system. Not finding it, she now wishes to look in other parts of the body. If there is no HIV in the T4 cells or the central nervous system of the other three AIDS patients, it must be somewhere else. Her next targets are the macrophages.

These are large cells which digest invading micro-organisms. They are found in the walls of blood vessels and some connective tissues. They interact with the T4 cells.

She said: 'We get higher percentages of virus recovery from macrophages than lymphocytes. When I started working on AIDS I too was asking how you get a virus which kills when it infects only one in 10,000 cells.

'Macrophages provide hormones which allow the lymphocytes to grow. The knowledge that macrophages with all their involvement in the other body systems are involved makes the relationship of HIV to AIDS much easier to understand.'

The requirement to inform the public, particularly in view of the seriousness of AIDS, is sometimes given for the reason why the 'HIV causes AIDS alone and with no other factor' theory was set in tablets of stone so quickly and then reinforced by government health warnings and a compliant media.

Of course the public had to be advised of the infectious nature of AIDS and the means of infection – intimate sexual contact, contaminated blood. They should have been told most emphatically about this long before the virus was isolated. The claim that the public need simplicity – to have an identifiable virus to associate with protective measures – is merely contemptuous of the public. In fact, the race to tell the public about the virus which was confused with the public health message was another part of the race for the prestige of discovery.

The public health message about condom use and abjuring shared syringes could have and should have been put into action in late 1982 when the transfusion cases made it certain that the disease was able to be transmitted by body cells. This had been a mainstream belief since 1981 but it would have been irresponsible to launch a public awareness programme then.

In fact there was no push for public awareness from the scientists – and countless thousands must have contracted the AIDS agent in the interim – until the battle for precedence in the discovery of HIV in 1984.

By this time the media were being told it was a public duty to inform all about the deadly virus. Any dissent on the issue of the cause of the disease was taken to be an undermining of the publicity campaign. In fact, the mechanism by which a disease is caused is almost always horrendously difficult to extrapolate while the means by which it is contracted is usually in little doubt. Non-A non-B hepatitis, for example, is caused by some unknown pathogen but its transmission and its effect on the body are well known. Similarly, we know the cause of almost no cancers at all but we know how they progress in the body. There is no contradiction in saying what we know but keeping quiet, or sharing our uncertainties, about what we do not know.

This public pressure, whether real or concocted, for a swift answer to the swiftly arrived problem of AIDS, was another pressure on the scientists which predisposed them to announce the success of a theory before it had been properly tested.

Partly by design, the discovery of HIV and the announcement that it caused AIDS was played out on a public platform. The deciding factors in whether this theory was to take precedence over all comers more closely resembled those in a court of law than a scientific debate. As in a court of law, where those who can afford the best counsel and who have tradition and authority on their side usually win, the HIV hypothesis won because the big labs and the big journals were backing it. As Montagnier said: 'I have learned more of politics than of science during all this. I never thought I would have to be a good salesman in order to be heard.'

State of the art

The act of observation alters that which is observed. Writing articles and making television programmes about a subject in the public domain must have some effect, or why do it?

The steady hammering on the inconsistencies in the HIV theory led to coverage in the general press, then the more popular scientific journals. By spring 1988 the *New Scientist*, *Science* and *Nature* had covered Duesberg's challenge to the AIDS establishment. Most serious newspapers in the US had covered it. Only the *New Scientist* presented a debate in which Duesberg put his points and a supporter of the HIV hypothesis responded. The film I and my collaborators made, *AIDS: The Unheard Voices*, had won the Royal Television Society Award for the best international current affairs programme of 1987.

Public pressure in the US for a hearing at which Peter Duesberg could debate his views before other scientists ended in a press meeting being called by the American Federation for AIDS Research in April 1988 at which no debate took place but five HIV supporters gave their views and Duesberg gave his.

Harry Rubin from Berkeley, another old hand at retrovirus work, was also present at this meeting. He keeps an open mind but argues for an appreciation of the complexity of biological systems in the face of Duesberg's challenge. He criticised the attitude of scientists who dismiss the challenge out of hand:

> It's all part of the hubris of modern molecular biology. These people think they have all the answers and the solution is just a matter of turning the crank. They believe in simple answers.
>
> Cartesian reductionism – the idea that all complex phenomena can be reduced to a molecule or a virus – doesn't make much sense in this situation. In biology there are too many people who go off half-cocked with all kinds of theories. We need to re-examine AIDS in the light of what Peter Duesberg is saying.

There are three propositions regarding HIV and its relationship with AIDS:

1. HIV is a deadly pathogen which kills fifty per cent or more of those infected. This is Robert Gallo's view.
2. HIV is a 'passenger' virus which is only mildly pathogenic; the cause of AIDS must be sought elsewhere. This is Peter Duesberg's view.
3. HIV is a necessary element of AIDS but will not cause the disease alone. It requires a susceptible host and/or another pathogen. This theory is rapidly gaining ground as the discrepancy between the number of people who have HIV infection and the number of people with AIDS increases.

Under Duesberg's onslaught, but without acknowledging him as the source of their discomfort, the supporters of the HIV theory are retreating from their original position. Once everyone said HIV got into T4 cells and killed them. Popular science magazines published diagrams on just how this happened. It was a Fact.

Now HIV supporters are vying to dream up new theories which will explain how HIV causes AIDS if it does not kill T4 cells directly. At the last count I knew of twelve. I have no intention of analysing theories about theories here.

It would indeed be a curse on both Gallo and Duesberg's houses if HIV does cause the disease but not in any way which Gallo proposed or which Duesberg contested.

Douglas McCormick, editor of the journal *Bio/Technology*, takes Duesberg's criticisms seriously. 'It may be time to re-evaluate the conventional wisdom,' he remarks. He suggests it is the protein envelope of the virus, not the genetic material of the virus itself, which is stimulating the body to shut down parts of its immune system. AIDS would be, therefore, an 'auto immune' disease – the body attacks itself.

AIDS has already offered us profound mysteries in addition to the mystery of its cause. John Crewdson, one of the most perceptive journalists who has written on AIDS listed these:

> Why do homosexual men with AIDS more often develop Kaposi's sarcoma rather than Pneumocystis carinii pneumonia, the most common opportunistic infection among other AIDS patients?
>
> Why does it take only about three years for many of those who have become infected with AIDS through transmissions of contaminated blood to get sick, compared with five years or more for many homosexual men who became infected through anal intercourse?
>
> Why are incubation times for children with AIDS shorter than for adults? Why are pipe smokers and men of British ancestry apparently at greater risk of acquiring AIDS than other men?

I am often urged, at meetings and in conversation, to give my own view of what causes AIDS. I am not a research scientist but my training in other fields tells me that the only wrong place to be is sitting on the fence: it is better to act and be wrong than to do nothing.

My view, informed only by literature on the subject and not by practical experience, is that HIV does not cause AIDS. Another pathogen, perhaps so far identified and perhaps not, is the causative agent. The situation is much complicated by the fact that the agent will cause AIDS only in those whose lifestyle predisposes them to immune deficiency or, perhaps, those who have a genetic predisposition to immune deficiency.

As to the question of where AIDS came from, I have not been greatly troubled as to where Lyme disease or tuberculosis or any other infectious condition came from, so I have been spared sleepless nights over my ignorance on the question of the origin of AIDS. I know that there are patterns of behaviour in which AIDS flourishes. Work on them seems a more appropriate use of resources than the attempt to pin down the point in space and time at which some hitherto harmless infectious agent mutated into a pathogen.

The future

It would be good to think the truth will out. In fact it is quite possible for medicine to proceed for many years with a theory which is wrong, giving treatments which are merely palliative.

It is also possible for adequate, successful treatments to be given which are successful despite their quite inaccurate theoretical basis.

One need not look to previous centuries for theories and treatments used long after their theoretical basis had been demolished – cupping and bleeding and the miasma and the humours. Examples abound in this century of 'scientific medicine'.

The treatment of diabetes with animal or synthetic insulin is a commonplace. It is a successful treatment and the scientist said to be its discoverer, Frederick Banting, enjoyed the accolade of the Nobel Prize in 1923. In fact, Banting's theoretical basis for his work on insulin was entirely wrong and his contribution to the production of usable insulin was minimal.

This is well described in Michael Bliss' book *The Discovery of Insulin*, a work of history published sixty years after the event. The weakness of Banting's theoretical base and his limited personal contribution should, one might think, have been appreciated earlier. As Bliss' researches uncovered, there had been a devastating and accurate criticism of Banting's hypothesis (and that of his research assistant Charles Best) by a Dr Ffrangcon Roberts in the *British Medical Journal* in 1922. After a lengthy paper Dr Roberts concluded that, though the work in Banting's lab led to insulin eventually, 'the production of insulin originated in a wrongly conceived, wrongly conducted and wrongly interpreted series of experiments.'

It was to no avail. Ffrangcon Roberts's criticism was put down to sour grapes (why hadn't *he* discovered insulin?) and in the medical textbooks in succeeding generations, right down to the present, the entirely inaccurate theoretical framework was passed on to medical students. They didn't question it either.

It is not entirely fair to make a direct connection between the discovery of HIV and the discovery of insulin, though points of comparison certainly exist. Most importantly, insulin actually worked. Diabetics were almost literally snatched from the grave. The hormone may have been purified for use by James Collip, a biochemist working near to Banting, but these men were in the same place at the same time and it was an effective treatment.

We will find out whether HIV causes AIDS but I predict this will happen a long way into the future and few will emerge from the historical record with much distinction.

As for the immediate future of the disease: the scenario does not look at all depressing for the mass of people who are not living intimately with a high-risk individual. The 'high risk' groups – homosexuals, intravenous drug users and haemophiliacs – still make up ninety per cent of AIDS cases in all areas where reporting can be said to be reasonably accurate. To be precise: in the US to 20 June 1988 it was ninety per cent. In the UK to the end of June 1988 it was ninety-three per cent. In the twenty-eight countries comprising the World Health

Organization surveillance report it was eighty-nine per cent to the end of December 1987.

Had we been in for big surprises – a massive increase in heterosexual cases, for example – we would have seen at least the beginning of the surprise in the first decade of the epidemic. To be more explicit: there should have been an increase in the number of heterosexual cases each month until they were taking a larger and larger percentage of the total number of cases. In fact, the percentage of heterosexual cases has stuck at four in the US and in the UK is statistically insignificant. There had been nine heterosexual AIDS cases in the UK up to the end of May 1988 who were said to have contracted the disease within the UK. This was the same as the number seven months previously. It is also the same as the number of people who died of cholera in England and Wales in a 1986 'mini-epidemic'. Proper precautions need to be taken if there is cholera, or AIDS, about, but let's not get carried away.

The continued preponderance of 'high risk' people in the AIDS figures strongly suggests it is something else these people do or have done to them, in addition to being infected with the 'AIDS agent', which causes their disease.

Of course, the fear is, for those who believe HIV causes AIDS, that there is a vast reservoir of AIDS-infected people who will develop the disease.

Looking at the figures for the US, which has long been taken as a model for AIDS in the rest of the world, it is obvious that the rate of increase in AIDS cases is slowing, despite that vast reservoir of HIV infection. In January 1982 it took five months for the number of AIDS cases to double. By May 1987 it had taken fourteen months for the most recent doubling. The numbers are big but a projection for the future, at least in the West, need not terrify.

In Africa, a good deal more clinical work needs to be done on the spread of AIDS and on establishing whether the cases currently identified as AIDS actually are identical with the cases identified in the West.

Some epidemics we live with, after all. TB is endemic in Africa, hepatitis B in Asia. Some epidemics whole populations live and die with. Diarrhoea kills five million children a year. The World Health Organization will have spent $1.5 billion on fighting AIDS by 1991, many times more than they have ever spent before or intend to spend in the future on diarrhoeal diseases.

Cervical cancer killed 2004 women in England and Wales in 1986. In the whole of the AIDS epidemic, up to the end of June 1988, AIDS had killed 897 people in the UK.

One scenario for the future would be of declining AIDS cases, caused by changes in lifestyle – homosexuals not engaging in the sort of behaviour which predisposes them to develop AIDS, intravenous drug users not sharing needles. This would be accompanied by the deaths of those not inclined to alter their behaviour. The epidemic would wear itself out in an ever-declining group of people doing risky things with their bodies.

It is conceivable that the disease itself could become less virulent, just as the syphilis which was the scourge of Europe, massively reducing its population in the sixteenth century, became the disease of the nineteenth century which took forty years to kill.

An example closer to today is that of scarlet fever. This was the scourge of childhood in the early part of this century, requiring quarantine and constant nursing for those who could afford it. The disease now causes a harmless rash which often goes unnoticed.

Improved treatments could increase the life expectancy of patients – there are already signs in the US that the case fatality rate (the number of AIDS cases who die) is in decline.

This could be a reporting error: physicians are reporting cases but not bothering later to report the deaths. This would be a surprising situation, as normally it occurs the other way around: the death figures are those which can be relied upon, not the cases.

There have been an increasing number of encouraging reports of people with AIDS living upwards of five years and living a normal life. Of almost 6000 people in New York with AIDS studied by the CDC, fifteen per cent were alive after five years. White homosexuals had done particularly well, with a third of them living after five years. A positive attitude and a healthy approach to life seem to be the most important factors in beating AIDS. If people consider a diagnosis of AIDS a sentence of death, for them it will be.

What should individuals who are HIV antibody-positive do? They should be using condoms in sex anyway, they should take care of themselves. But as Peter Duesberg said: 'Being HIV-antibody positive is not something to commit suicide for, or burn someone's house down over.'

Even if I am wrong and HIV does cause AIDS, it is an extremely difficult disease to contract. Tolerance is a particular virtue when we feel endangered. We could use more of it.

AIDS has become the greatest fear for many people who are at no risk whatsoever. It is difficult to give reassurance when fears are so irrational but, remember, we represent a long, long period of evolution. Don't be frightened. We are going to live.

Abbreviations

Abbreviations have been kept to a minimum. Wherever, in the early days of its life, HIV was being referred to as LAV, HTLV-III or any of its other names, I have altered this to HIV which was the nomenclature agreed on internationally in May 1986. The only exception to this is Chapter 3 where the earlier names are used when appropriate.

For ease of reading, micro-organisms which are normally italicised do not have that treatment in this text except in the index.

The original HIV is referred to as HIV-1 only when a direct comparison is made with HIV-2.

AIDS	Acquired Immune Deficiency Syndrome
CDC	Centers for Disease Control, Atlanta, Georgia, USA
DNA	Deoxyribonucleic Acid – the complex chemical which encodes basic genetic information. Present in body cells of all living things including 'DNA viruses'.
HIV	Human Immunodeficiency Virus
HTLV-I	Human T-cell Leukaemia Virus I
HTLV-II	Human T-cell Leukaemia Virus II
HTLV-III	Human T-cell Lymphotropic Virus III
NIH	National Institutes of Health, Bethesda, Maryland, USA
LAV	Lymphadenopathy-Associated Virus
RNA	Ribonucleic Acid – replaces DNA as a carrier of genetic codes in some viruses including retroviruses. Controls protein synthesis in all living cells

It can be taken that everyone quoted is a scientist unless otherwise mentioned. Some journalists are quoted, for example. It is simpler not to give titles when there is a confusion between the 'doctor' who has a medical degree and the 'doctor' who does not. Additionally, the term 'professor' can confer a quite different level of seniority from one side of the Atlantic to another. All people quoted have academic backgrounds which make their comments tenable.

One error made throughout, with regret, is the description of AIDS as 'the disease'. It is not, of course, a single disease but a syndrome, a collection of diseases which indicate an underlying immune deficiency.

Notes

Beginnings

Adams, J., and Verney-Elliott, M., 'AIDS – The Unheard Voices', *Dispatches*, Channel 4, 13 November 1987.

Patients

Fettner, A.G., and Check, W., *The Truth About AIDS*, New York, 1985. Invaluable source material on early events. Picture of Gottlieb particularly indebted to Fettner and Check.

Cahill, K.M., *The AIDS Epidemic*, London 1984.

Cantwell, A., *AIDS: The Mystery and the Solution*, Los Angeles, 1986.

Gong, V., and Rudnick, N., *AIDS: Facts and Issues*, London, 1986.

Siegel, F.P., and Siegel, M., *AIDS: The Medical Mystery*, New York, 1983.

Wellcome Foundation Limited. *New Perspectives on Herpes Virus Infections* (press conference document), London, 1986.

Javier, R.T., Sedarati, F., and Stevens, J.G., 'Two Avirulent Herpes Simplex Viruses Generate Lethal Recombinations in Vitro', *Science* 234, 1986, pp. 746–7.

Beldekas, J., Teas, J., and Herbert, J.R., 'African Swine Fever Virus and Aids', *Lancet*, 8 March 1986, pp. 564–5.

Lo, S.C., 'Isolation and Identification of a Novel Virus from Patients With AIDS', *American Journal of Tropical Medicine and Hygiene*, July 1986, pp. 675–6.

Lo, S.C., *et al.*, 'A Newly Identified Virus-Like Infectious Agent Derived from a Patient with AIDS', abstract presented at Fourth International Conference on AIDS, Stockholm, June 1988.

Lo, S.C., *et al.*, 'Fatal Infection of Non-Human Primates with the Virus-like Infectious Agent (VLIA-sb51) Derived From a Patient with AIDS', abstract presented at Fourth International Conference on AIDS, Stockholm, June 1988. Both abstracts available from Armed Forces Institute of Pathology, Washington, DC.

Ostrom, N., 'Chronic Fatigue Report', *New York Native*, 4 April 1988.

Crown, S., 'Personal View', *British Medical Journal* 294, 1987, p. 1349.

McAnally, C., *AIDS: A Priest's Testament*, Channel 4 TV, 8 November 1987.

Centers for Disease Control, *AIDS Weekly Surveillance Report*.

Farber, C., 'AIDS: Words from the Front', *Spin*, June 1988.

Stewart, G., 'Limitations of the Germ Theory', *Lancet*, 18 May 1968, p. 1077.

'No Need for Panic About AIDS', unsigned article, *Nature* 302, 1983, p. 749.

Lifson, A.R., *et al.*, 'The Epidemiology of AIDS Worldwide', *Clinics in Immunology & Allergy*, October 1986, pp. 441–65.

Rubinstein, A., 'Children with AIDS and the Public Risk', Gong and Rudnik, op. cit.

Seale, J., 'An AIDS Challenge on the Dangers of Kissing', *Guardian*, 20 January 1987.

Salahuddin, S.Z., *et al.*, 'HTLV-III in Symptom-Free Seronegative Persons', *Lancet*, 22/29 December 1984, pp. 1418–20.

Salahuddin, S.Z., *et al.*, 'Isolation of a new virus, HBLV, in Patients with Lymphoproliferative Disorders', *Science* 234, 1986, pp. 596–601.

Ho, D.D., *et al.*, 'Infrequency of Isolation of HTLV-III virus from Saliva in AIDS', *New England Journal of Medicine*, 19 December 1985, p. 1606.

Groopman, J.E., *et al.*, 'HTLV-III in Saliva of People with AIDS-related Complex and Healthy Homosexual Men at Risk for AIDS', *Science* 224, 1984, pp. 500–3.

Acheson, D., 'Carry on Kissing', *Guardian*, 30 January 1987.

Monckton, C., 'Concern for the Kiss', *Guardian*, 3 February 1987.

Smith, J.W.G., 'HIV Transmitted by Sexual Intercourse but not by Kissing', *British Medical Journal* 294, 1987, p. 446.

Wahn, V., *et al.*, 'Horizontal Transmission of HIV Infection Between Two Siblings', *Lancet*, 20 September 1986, p. 694.

Ho, D.D., *et al.*, 'HTLV-III in the Semen and Blood of a Healthy Homosexual Man', *Science* 226, 1984, pp. 447–9.

Zagury, D., *et al.*, 'HTLV-III in Cells Cultured from Semen of Two Patients With AIDS', *Science* 226, 1984, pp. 449–51.

Kay, L.A., and Griffiths, R.K., 'If Scientists Lose their Heads Over AIDS', *Guardian*, 4 February 1987.

Rawlins, J., 'AIDS and the Heterosexual Epidemic', *British Medical Journal* 294, 1987, p. 970.

Monzon, O.T., and Capellan, J.M.B., 'Female to Female Transmission of HIV', *Lancet*, 4 July 1987.

Calabrese, L.H., and Gopalakrishna, K.V., 'Transmission of HTLV-III Infection from Man to Woman to Man', *New England Journal of Medicine* 314, 1986, p. 987.

Virus Hunters

Dulbecco, R., *Francis Peyton Rous*, Washington, 1976.

Much of the sheer fact is from standard works of reference on general medicine, in particular Weatherall, D.J. (ed.), *Oxford Textbook of Medicine*, Oxford, 1987.

Bailar, J.C., and Smith, E.M., 'Progress Against Cancer?', *New England Journal of Medicine*, 8 May 1986, pp. 1226–32.

Cairns, J., 'The Treatment of Diseases and the War Against Cancer', *Scientific American*, November 1985, pp. 51–9.

Gallo, R.C., 'The First Human Retrovirus', *Scientific American*, December 1986, pp. 88–98.

Remnick, D., 'Robert Gallo Goes to War', *Washington Post*, 9 August 1987. A classic of adulatory journalism.

Gallo, R.C., 'HTLV-III: Untangling the Retroviral Origin of the AIDS Pandemic', *Advances in Oncology*, Vol. 2, No. 3, 1986, pp. 3–10.

Duesberg, P., 'Retroviruses as Carcinogens and Pathogens: Expectations and Reality', *Cancer Research*, 1 March 1987, pp. 1199–220.

Shilts, R., *And the Band Played On*, New York, 1987.

Connor, Steve, 'AIDS: Science Stands on Trial', *New Scientist*, 12 February 1987, pp. 49–58. Easily the best history written on this early period of research and the battle between Gallo's lab and Montagnier's. This chapter is much indebted to it.

Connor, Steve, 'AIDS: Mystery of the Missing Data', *New Scientist*, 12 February, p. 19.

Black, David, op. cit.

Gilden, Raymond V., 'HTLV-III Legend Corrected', *Science*, 18 April 1986, p. 307.

'Why the AIDS virus is not like HTLVs I or II', unsigned article in *New Scientist*, 7 February 1985, p. 4.

Some issues – naming of the virus, settling of the dispute between Gallo and Montagnier – are so clearly in the public domain that they are not referenced.

Koch, M., 'The Anatomy of the Virus', *New Scientist*, 26 March 1987, pp. 46–51.

'In Pursuit of AIDS', editorial in *New Scientist*, 7 February 1985.

Burgdorfer, W., 'Lyme Disease – a Tick Borne Spirochetosis?', *Science* 216, 1982, pp. 1317–19.

Cantwell, A., op. cit.

Sarkur, N.H., 'Type B Virus and Human Breast Cancer', *The Role of Viruses in Human Cancer*, Giraldo, G., and Beth, E. (eds), Amsterdam, 1980, pp. 206–33.

Al-Sumidaie, A.M., *et al.*, 'Particles with Properties of Retroviruses in Monocytes from Patients with Breast Cancer', *Lancet*, 2/9 January 1988, pp. 5–9.

Iwarson, S.A., 'Non-A, Non-B Hepatitis: Dead Ends or New Horizons?', *British Medical Journal*, 17 October 1987, pp. 946–8.

Shulman, S.T., and Rowley, A.H., 'Does Kawasaki Disease Have a Retroviral Aetiology?', *Lancet*, 6 September 1986, pp. 545–6.

Monmaney, T., *et al.*, 'Another AIDS Virus Appears', *Newsweek*, 11 January 1988, pp. 46–7.

Clavel, F., *et al.*, 'Isolation of a New Human Retrovirus from West African Patients with AIDS', *Science* 233, 1986, pp. 343–6.

Kanki, P.J., Alroy, J., and Essex, M., 'Isolation of T-Lymphotropic Retrovirus Related to HTLV-III/LAV from Wild-Caught African Green Monkeys', *Science* 230, 1985, pp. 951–4.

Albert, J., *et al.*, 'A New Human Retrovirus Isolate of West African Origin (SBL-6669) and Its Relationship to HTLV-I, LAV and HTLV-IIIB', *AIDS and Human Retrovirus Research*, Spring 1987, pp. 3–10.

Desrosiers, R.C., *et al.*, 'Origins of HTLV-4', *Nature* 327, 1987, p. 107.

Manzari, V., 'HTLV-V: A New Human Retrovirus Isolated in a Tac-Negative T-Cell Lymphoma/Leukaemia', *Science*, 11 December 1987.

Newmark, P., and Anderson, A., 'AIDS Conference Launched with Controversial Message', *Nature* 327,1987, p. 355.

AIDS Research, Vol. 2, No. 4, 1986.

AIDS Research and Human Retroviruses, Vol. 3, No. 1, 1987.

Kingman, S., and Connor, S., '"Third" AIDS virus unveiled at Stockholm', *New Scientist*, 16 June 1988.

HIV Challenged

Gallo, R.C., Introduction for P.H. Duesberg, *Haematology and Blood Transfusion*, Vol. 29, *Modern Trends in Human Leukaemia VI*, Neth, Gallo, Greaves, Janka (eds), Berlin, 1985, pp. 7–8.

Duesberg, R.C., 'Cancer Research', op. cit.

Von Briesen, H., Rübsamen-Waigmann, H., *et al.*, 'Isolation Frequency and Growth Properties of HIV-Variants: Multiple Simultaneous Variants in a Patient Demonstrated by Molecular Cloning', *Journal of Medical Virology* 23, 1987, pp. 51–66. This paper does not give the figures quoted (of ninety-one patients, three failed to yield up virus) but Helga Rübsamen-Waigmann told Peter Duesberg this was the case, as quoted in the *Cancer Research* paper, and repeated it to me on 8 February 1988. The only clear figure this paper gives is that HIV could be isolated from only 80 per cent of AIDS cases. This is particularly significant considering the sensitivity of the equipment used and the high standards of the lab work.

Lauritsen, J., 'Saying No to HIV', *New York Native*, 6 July 1987, pp. 17–25.

Walker, C.M., *et al.*, 'CD8+ Lymphocytes Can Control HIV Infection in Vitro by Suppressing Virus Replication', *Science* 234, 1986, pp. 1563–6.

Shaw, G.M., *et al.*, 'Molecular Characterisation of Human T-Cell Leukaemia (Lymphotropic) Virus Type III in the Acquired Immune Deficiency Syndrome', *Science* 226, 1984, pp. 1165–71.

'Leads From the MMWR', unsigned article in *Journal of the American Medical Association*, 4 September 1987, p. 1149.

Gong, op. cit., *Facts and Fallacies: An AIDS Overview*.

'Revised Case Definition of AIDS', unsigned article in *British Medical Journal*, 31 October 1987, p. 1125.

AIDS Weekly Surveillance Reports from United States AIDS Program, Center for Infectious Diseases, Centers for Disease Control.

AIDS Surveillance in Europe, Quarterly Reports, WHO Collaborating Centre on AIDS.

Centers for Disease Control, *Morbidity and Mortality Weekly Report*, Vol. 34, June 1985, p. 375.

Le Fanu, J., *Eat Your Heart Out – The Rise and Fall of the Healthy Diet*, London, 1987.

Farber, C., 'AIDS. Words From the Front', *Spin*, January 1988.

Liversidge, A., 'AIDS. Words From the Front', *Spin*, February 1988.

'New definition inflates figures', unsigned article in *New Scientist*, 12 May 1988.

Centers for Disease Control, 'AIDS and HIV Infection Among Health-Care Workers', *Vol. 37*, April 1988, pp. 229–39.

Five Hs

Ingram, G.I.C., 'The History of Haemophilia', *Journal of Clinical Pathology* 29, 1976, pp. 469–79.

Johnson, R.E., *et al.*, 'Acquired Immunodeficiency Syndrome Among Patients Attending Hemophilia Treatment Centers and Mortality Experience of Hemophiliacs in the United States', *American Journal of Epidemiology* 121, 1985, pp. 797–810.

Rock, A., 'Inside the Billion-Dollar Business of Blood', *Money*, March 1986, pp. 153–72. A fine work of journalism.

Ablin, R.J., 'Transglutaminase: Co-Factor in Aetiology of AIDS?', *Lancet*, 6 April 1985, pp. 813–14.

Ablin, R.J., 'A Noninfectious Copathogenesis of AIDS', *Clinical Immunology Newsletter*, August 1987, pp. 127–8.

Hoggart, S., 'The Fall of the House of Papa Doc', *Observer*, 9 February 1986.

Fettner, op. cit.

Gong, op. cit.

Pape, J.W., 'Characteristics of the Acquired Immunodeficiency Syndrome in Haiti', *New England Journal of Medicine* 309, 1983, pp. 945–9.

Cahill, K.M., op. cit.

Hutchinson, R., 'Heroin: A Political Fix', *Time Out*, 8 August 1975, pp. 11–15.

Moss, A.R., 'AIDS and Intravenous Drug Use: The Real Heterosexual Epidemic', *British Medical Journal*, 14 February 1987, pp. 389–90.

Krieger, T., and Caceres, C.A., 'The Unnoticed Link in AIDS Cases', *Wall Street Journal*, 24 October 1985.

Altman, D., *Homosexual Oppression and Liberation*, London, 1974.

Kramer, L., *Faggots*, New York, 1978.

Sexual pleasure in ancient times had been inadequately researched with the exception of that of the Romans about which we know a great deal, doubtless at the expense of studies of other great civilisations. Aries, P., and Duby, G., *A History of Private Life from Pagan Rome to Byzantium*, London, 1987, goes some way to redressing this. A lubricious account of the sexual pleasures of the Chinese court is given in Chou, E., *The Dragon and the Phoenix*, London, 1971.

Rist, D. Yates, 'Dying for our Fantasies', *The Volunteer* 4, 1987, p. 1.

Rist, D. Yates, 'Policing the Libido', *Village Voice*, 26 November 1985.

Rist, D. Yates, 'AIDS and Axelrod's Bad Medicine: One Way to Kill Off Straights', *New York Native*, 23 December 1985.

Kramer, L., '1112 and Counting', *New York Native*, 7 March 1983.

Shilts, R., op. cit.

Lauritsen, J., and Wilson, H., *Death Rush – Poppers and AIDS*, San Francisco, 1986.

Luzi, G., 'Transmission of HTLV-III Infection by Heterosexual Contact', *Lancet*, 2 November 1985, p. 1018.

Papaevangelou, G., 'LAV/HTLV-III Infection in Female Prostitutes', *Lancet*, 2 November 1985, p. 1018.

Barton, S.E., 'HTLV-III Antibody in Prostitutes', *Lancet*, 21/28 December 1985, p. 1424.

Tirelli, U., 'HTLV-III Antibody in Prostitutes', *Lancet*, 21/28 December 1985, p. 1424.

Smith, G.L., 'Lack of HIV Infection and Condom Use in Licensed Prostitutes', *Lancet*, 13 December 1986, p. 1392.

'Shared Needles Spread AIDS to Heterosexuals and Heterosexual AIDS Comes to Britain', unsigned article in *New Scientist*, 11 June 1987, p. 27.

Associated Press tapes, 'Anti-AIDS Crusader Sommatra Troy Criticises Australian News Report Describing Thailand as "AIDS Capital" of Southeast Asia', 1 November 1987.

Associated Press tapes, 'Nearly 100 People Found to Be Carrying the AIDS Virus in Thailand', 17 July 1987.

'Condoms Come to the Rescue in Thailand', unsigned article in *New Scientist*, 21 January 1988, pp. 28–9.

Sun-Han, K., 'Korean Doctor Dedicates Herself to Crusade Against VD', *Bangkok Post*, 31 December 1987.

Anderson, speaking in 'AIDS Now: Is There Going to Be a Heterosexual Epidemic?', Channel 4 TV (UK), 5 February 1988.

Syphilis

Coulter, H.L., *AIDS and Syphilis – The Hidden Link*, Berkeley, 1987. An invaluable alternative view of AIDS. Some parts of this chapter rely heavily on it, in particular the references to Stephen Caiazza's first contact with Joan McKenna and Klaus-Uwe Dierig, where Stephen Caiazza assured me that Coulter's account was entirely accurate so I did not bother him with a request to repeat it.

Felstein, F., *Sexual Pollution*, Newton Abbot, 1974.

Major, R.H., *A History of Medicine*, Oxford, 1954.

Cherniak, D., and Feingold, A., *VD Handbook*, Montreal, 1972.

Csonka, G.W., 'Syphilis', in *Oxford Textbook of Medicine*, Oxford, 1987. Once again a debt is due to these splendid volumes.

Hooshmand, H., *et al.*, 'Neurosyphilis: a Study of 241 Patients', *Journal of the American Medical Association* 219, 1972, p. 726.

Johnson, C., 'One Epidemic or Two? The Syphilis/AIDS Connection', *New York Native*, 4 May 1987, pp. 13–20.

Poulsen, A., 'Regression of Kaposi's Sarcoma in AIDS After Treatment with Dapsone', *Lancet*, 10 March 1984, p. 560.

Faber, V., 'Inhibition of HIV Replication In Vitro by Fusidic Acid', *Lancet*, 10 October 1987, pp. 827–8.

Burgdorfer, op. cit.

'Possible Link Between Syphilis and AIDS', unsigned article in *New Scientist*, 30 April 1987, p. 30.

Origins

Cahill, Kevin M., *The AIDS Epidemic*, London, 1984. Untainted source of material on the early clinical manifestations of AIDS and early ideas of its cause.

Hoyle, F., and Wickramasinghe, N.C., *Nature* 327, 1987, p. 664.

Hoyle, F., and Wickramasinghe, N.C., *Diseases from Space*, London, 1979. On the general theory.

Veitch, A., '"AIDS Created" Claim Renewed', *Guardian*, 27 October 1986.

Seale, J., Letter to the *Journal of the Royal Society of Medicine*, August 1986, pp. 494–5.

Black, D., *The Plague Years*, London, 1986.

Ortleb, C., 'The AIDS Explosion in Cuba', *New York Native*, 17 February 1986.

Cumulative AIDS Cases as Reported to WHO as of 12 January 1988. Document available for World Summit of Ministers of Health on Programmes for AIDS Prevention, London, January 1988.

Many of the more outlandish conspiracy theories are anecdotal in nature – they do not bear too much writing down and are not able to be fully referenced. If they could be, they would not, of course, be conspiracy theories.

Teas, J., 'Could AIDS Agent Be a New Variant of African Swine Fever Virus?', *Lancet*, 23 April 1983, p. 923.

Beldekas, J.C., *et al.*, 'In Vitro Effect of Foscarnet on Expansion of T-Cells from People with LAV and AIDS', *Lancet*, 16 November 1985, pp. 1128–9.

'Jane Teas Urges Senator Kennedy to Begin Swine Fever Inquiry', *New York Native*, 30 September 1985.

Beldekas, J., Teas, J., and Herbert, J.R., 'African Swine Fever Virus and AIDS', *Lancet*, 8 March 1986, pp. 564–5.

Leishman, K., 'AIDS and Insects', *Atlantic Monthly*, September 1987, pp. 56–72.

'Pigs, AIDS and Belle Glade', *New York Times*, 3 June 1986.

Associated Press tapes, 8 March 1986.

Discussions with and practical help from John Beldekas and Jane Teas have been invaluable.

Redfield, Robert R., *et al.*, 'Disseminated Vaccinia in a Military Recruit with Human Immunodeficiency Virus (HIV) Disease', *New England Journal of Medicine*, 12 March 1987, pp. 673–6.

Wright, P., 'Smallpox Vaccine "Triggered AIDS Virus"' *The Times*, 11 May 1987.

Veitch, A., 'Smallpox Blame for AIDS Dismissed', *Guardian*, 12 May 1987.

Delarue, S., 'Role des vaccinations dans la transmission et le déclenchement du sida', *Santé Liberté et Vaccinations*, Octobre, Novembre, Decembre 1987, pp. 2–8.

Kanki, P.J., Alroy, J., and Essex, M., 'Isolation of T-Lymphotropic Retrovirus Related to HTLV-III/LAV from Wild Caught African Green Monkeys', *Science* 230, 1985, pp. 951–4.

Clavel, F., *et al.*, 'Isolation of a New Human Retrovirus from West African Patients with AIDS', *Science* 233, 1986, pp. 343–6.

Karpas, A., 'Origin of the AIDS Virus Explained?', *New Scientist*, 16 July 1987, p. 67.

'The Monkey's Blood', unsigned article, *The Economist*, 25 July 1987, p. 76.

Giunta, S., and Groppa, G., 'The Primate Trade and the Origin of AIDS Viruses', *Nature* 329, 1987, p. 22.

Creamer, J. (ed.), *Biohazard – The Silent Threat from Biomedical Research and the Creation of AIDS*, London, 1987.

Jones, P., 'AIDS – The African Connection?', *British Medical Journal*, 20 July 1985, p. 216.

Hagen, Piet, *Blood – Gift or Merchandise?*, New York, 1982. This book is the starting point for all investigations of international blood dealing.

'American Boy Died of AIDS 18 Years Ago', *Daily Telegraph*, 26 October 1987.

Stewart, G.T., 'A Study of the Factors Associated with Addiction to Heroin', *Report to the National Institute of Mental Health* RO1 Mh 18229 (1/70–12/71).

Stoneburner, R.L., *et al.*, 'Increasing Mortality Among Intravenous Drug Users in New York City and its Relationship to the AIDS Epidemic: Evidence for a Larger Spectrum of HIV-Related Disease'. Presented to American Public Health Association 115th Annual Meeting, New Orleans, 18–22 October 1987.

McFarlane, R., Letter in *The Volunteer* (Gay Men's Health Crisis Newsletter), Vol. 4, No. 2, 1987.

Medicaid information for New York City accurate in 1984 when I did the research for *Who Cares?*, a series of television programmes on health care in different countries, Channel 4 (UK), 17 May 1985, and for four following weeks.

Africa

'AIDS and the Third World', *Panos Dossier* 1, London, 1986.

Chirimuuta, R.C., and Chirimuuta, R.J., *Aids, Africa and Racism*, Bretby, 1987.

Konotey-Ahulu, F.I.D., 'AIDS in Africa: Misinformation and Disinformation', *Lancet*, 25 July 1987, pp. 206–7. Many thanks to Konotey-Ahulu for his consistent sanity and correspondence.

Konotey-Ahulu, F.I.D., 'Clinical Epidemiology, Not Seroepidemiology, Is the Answer to Africa's AIDS Problem', *British Medical Journal*, 20 June 1987, pp. 1593–4.

Ochieng, P., 'Africa Not to Blame for AIDS', *New African*, January 1987, p. 25.

Nahmias, A.J., 'Evidence for Human Infection with an HTLV-III/LAV-Like Virus in Central Africa, 1959', *Lancet*, 31 May 1986, pp. 1279–80.

Mann, J., 'AIDS in Africa', *New Scientist*, 26 March 1987, pp. 40–3.

Wendler, I., 'Seroepidemiology of Human Immunodeficiency Virus in Africa', *British Medical Journal*, 27 September 1986, pp. 782–5.

'Evidence for Origin Is Weak', unsigned article in *New Scientist*, 15 October 1987, p. 27.

Connor, S., 'Monkey Diet "May Hold Key to AIDS Cure"', *New Scientist*, 17 December 1987.

'The confusing case of African AIDS', unsigned article in *New Scientist*, 18 February 1988.

Connor, S., and Kingman, S., *The Search for the Virus*, London, 1988.

Money

'Gallo to Stay at NIH – For Now, at Least', *Science*, 4 December 1987, p. 1349.

Farber, C., op. cit.

Technology Management Group, *World Market for AIDS Drugs, Vaccines and Diagnostics Projected to Exceed $3 Billion by 1996*, Stamford, Connecticut, 29 July 1986.

Weisberg, M.S., 'AIDS: The New Money-Maker', *Daily News*, New York, 18 August 1987.

US Budget figures: Associated Press tapes.

Karpas, A., *et al.*, 'Lytic Infection by British AIDS Virus and Development of Rapid Cell Test for Antiviral Antibodies', *Lancet*, 28 September 1985, pp. 695–7.

Price, L., 'Scientists' squabbles "may have cost lives"', *Listener*, 26 February 1987, p. 7.

Karpas, A., 'AIDS and HIV', *Listener*, 7 January 1988, p. 20.

Connor, S., 'Japan buys British "litmus test" for AIDS', *New Scientist*, 28 August 1986, p. 18.

Rees, D.A., 'AIDS and HIV', *Listener*, 11 February 1988, p. 18.

Mazzitelli, T., 'AIDS Profits Take Off "Like Any Other Business"', *Gemini News Service*, 20 November 1987.

Jackson, T., 'Gambling on AIDS Drug Gives Wellcome a Happy Anniversary', *Financial Times*, 21 February 1987.

Erlichman, J., 'Welcoming some nice, easy profits from AIDS monopoly', *Guardian*, 23 October 1987.

'The awful cost of AIDS', unsigned article in *The Economist*, 11 April 1987, pp. 31–2.

Fischl, M.A., *et al.*, 'The Efficacy of Azidothymidine (AZT) in the Treatment of Patients with AIDS and AIDS-Related Complex', *New England Journal of Medicine*, 23 July 1987, pp. 185–97.

Azidothymidine – A Potential Treatment for AIDS, Public Relations Department, The Wellcome Foundation Limited, 5 November 1986.

Zidovudine – What It Is, Kingsway Public Relations (for Wellcome), London, 23 September 1987.

Retrovir Capsules (Zidovudine), Data Sheet, Burroughs Wellcome Co., USA, 1987.

'Zidovudine (AZT)', unsigned article in *Lancet*, 25 April 1987, pp. 957–8.

'Link with Syphilis Grows Stronger', unsigned article in *New Scientist*, 6 August 1987, p. 24.

Farber, C., 'AIDS – Words from the Front', *Spin*, December 1987, pp. 73–5.

'Harvard patents the coat of the AIDS virus', unsigned article in *New Scientist*, 25 February 1988.

Lauritsen, J., 'AZT on Trial', *New York Native*, 19 October 1987.

Endgame

Feyerabend, P., *Against Method*, London, 1978.

Weber, J., 'AIDS and the "guilty" virus', *New Scientist*, 5 May 1988.

McCormick, D., 'Beyond Buzzwords in AIDS Pathogenesis', *Biotechnology*, December 1987, p. 1249.

Rapoport, R., 'Dissident Scientist's AIDS Theory Angers Colleagues', *Sunday Tribune*, Oakland, California, 31 January 1988.

UK death figures for other diseases from Office of Population, Census and Surveys, London.

Crewdson, J., 'AIDS Prognosis Still Elusive', *Chicago Tribune*, 31 May 1987.

Crewdson, J., 'Studies hint AIDS spread less severe than predicted', *Chicago Tribune*, 1 June 1987.

Buchanan, P.J., widely syndicated column, 24 May 1983.

Bliss, M., *The Discovery of Insulin*, Toronto, 1982.

Index